Care of the Professional Voice

The colour plates used in this book were made possible through a grant made by the Handel Evans family in memory of Dr Handel Parry Evans (Mus Doc) who devoted his life to music and in particular the encouragement and training of young singers

Care of the Professional Voice:

A Management Guide for Singers, Actors and Professional Voice Users

D. Garfield Davies MB BS FRCS Hon FRAM
Consultant Emeritus Otolaryngologist to The Middlesex and University College Hospitals (UCL Hospitals)
Laryngologist to the Vocal Faculty Royal Academy of Music, Trinity College of Music, the Royal Shakespeare Company, the London Academy for Music and Dramatic Art, the Royal National Theatre, the English National Opera and the Royal Opera House

ERRATUM

Anthony F. Jahn MD FACS FRCS (C)
Professor of Clinical Otolaryngology, Columbia University College of Physicians and Surgeons, New York
Director of Otolaryngology, The Miller Institute for Performing Arts Medicine, New York
Adjunct Professor of Vocal Pedagogy, Westminster Choir College, Princeton, New Jersey
Adjunct Professor of Neurosciences, Rutgers University, Newark, New Jersey

BUTTERWORTH HEINEMANN

OXFORD   BOSTON   JOHANNESBURG   MELBOURNE   NEW DELHI   SINGAPORE

Butterworth-Heinemann
Linacre House, Jordan Hill, Oxford OX2 8DP
225 Wildwood Avenue, Woburn, MA 01801-2041
A division of Reed Educational and Professional Publishing Ltd

℞ A member of the Reed Elsevier plc group

First published 1998

British Library Cataloguing in Publication Data
Care of the professional voice: a management guide for
   singers, actors and professional voice users
   1. Voice – Care and hygiene   2. Singing
   612.7'8'024782

ISBN 0 7506 3640 8

Library of Congress Cataloguing in Publication Data
Davies, D. Garfield.
   Care of the professional voice: a management guide for singers,
   actors, and professional voice users/D. Garfield Davies, Anthony
   F. Jahn.
   p. cm.
   Includes bibliographical references and index.
   ISBN 0 7506 3640 8
   1. Voice – Care and hygiene.   2.   Voice – Physiological aspects.
   3. Singers – Health and hygiene.   4. Actors – Health and hygiene.
   5. Voice disorders.   I. Jahn, Anthony F.   II. Title.
   RF511.S55D38   98–22187
   616.85'5–dc21   CIP

Photoset by Wilmaset Ltd, Birkenhead, Wirral
Printed and bound in Great Britain by Biddles Ltd, Guildford and Kings Lynn

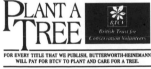

Contents

Foreword

At last! A brief, well-illustrated, easy to understand medical reference for anyone dependent on their voice.

In addition to a discussion of vocal anatomy and disorders, this book contains useful information on matters such as travelling, environmental effects and medications. These subjects are as much a part of a singer's life as the actual performance.

Along with their medical credentials, the authors bring to this book years of personal experience in the theatre – I have personally consulted with both of them on many occasions, and their advice has proven invaluable.

This volume should become a staple of every singer/actor's library.

James Morris
Metropolitan Opera, New York

Anyone whose voice is their livelihood will welcome this succinct and user-friendly book. We know how important it is that we look after our voices and this illustrated book offers practical medical information and insight that will be of great use to individuals and academics alike.

I expect it to become a valuable handbook for all manner of vocal performers and I am delighted to commend it to you.

Sir Anthony Hopkins

Preface

Singers and actors constitute a unique group of performers. Relying almost entirely on their voice for their livelihood, these artists work in a stressful and highly competitive environment. As the twentieth century draws to a close, the life of the vocal performer grows ever more hectic and demanding. In addition to problems intrinsic to singing, the singer or actor must also cope with jet lag, electronic enhancement and an ever-increasing number of allergens and pollutants in the performing environment. Other professional voice users such as lawyers, teachers, politicians and public speakers are also exposed to a hectic life and experience many of the problems encountered by the professional vocal artist.

There are numerous books available to laryngologists with an interest in the voice. There is, however, a lack of literature which ties together laryngology with the many related issues faced by both vocal artists and their physicians working together in the business of vocal performing arts. While many physicians treat singers and actors, we believe that optimal treatment can only be given if the doctor understands not only the medical problem but also the patient, the vocal task, and the working milieu, whether opera, popular theatre or legitimate stage.

In writing this book, our original plan was to update Norman Punt's classic volume *The Singer's and Actor's Throat*. That book, now out of print, was unique in that it attempted to speak to both the physician and the vocal professional. As we began our task, it became clear that enormous changes have taken place both in the field of vocal performance as well as in the field of laryngology; changes which called for an entirely new book, rather than just a revision.

While the book is new, we have tried to keep within the spirit of Punt's work. The volume is small, portable, and attempts to bring together both vocalist and physician on common ground.

Although the two professions share a common interest, there are clearly chapters which speak to one group more than the other. We apologize if some of the terms and concepts are more technical than other parts, but we trust that the short glossary provided will aid understanding. We hope that the patience and persistence demanded by these chapters will be rewarded through the expansion of shared knowledge, to the benefit of the greatest of instruments, the human voice.

D. Garfield Davies
London
Anthony F. Jahn
New York

Acknowledgements

We would like to thank the following for supplying the illustrations for this book: Martin Dunitz and Professor Bruce Benjamin (Plates 6, 7, 8, 9, 11 and 15), Dr Steve Zeitels (Plate 10a) and Jean Abitbol (Plates 10b, 12, 13 and 14).

We would also like to acknowledge Anat Keidar PhD for insights into the links between physiology and psychology of the singing voice; Robert Bastian MD for collegial advice on vocal fold surgery, and the late Eugen Grabscheid MD for imparting his mastery of the art of working with singers.

We are also grateful to Christina Shewell and Ruth Epstein, voice therapists par excellence for their great help and advice over the years. In addition we are indebted to the Mackintosh Trust for their support in helping to make this publication possible.

Anatomy and physiology of the vocal mechanism

Introduction

When we consider the anatomical parts relevant to the voice, we naturally think of the larynx. The larynx, or voice box, is a highly specialized organ which is perched on top of the trachea (windpipe), and acts as the sound source generator during phonation or singing. There are, however, other equally important anatomical structures above and below the larynx, without which the voice could not be produced. These include the mouth, the palate, the pharynx and the lower airway (trachea, bronchi and lungs), as well as the abdomen and even the pelvis. In fact, there are only a few parts of the body not involved in some way in the process of voice production.

Let us now consider the entire vocal tract, and 'follow the voice' from its beginnings to its full formation.

The thorax and abdomen

The energy powering the voice is air which is exhaled from the lungs. The lungs are passive bellows within the thoracic cage, which inflate on inspiration and deflate on expiration. The thoracic cage is a rather rigid compartment with a flexible floor: the diaphragm. This thin partition of muscle and fibrous tissue forms a dome which is convex upward (thoracic aspect), and concave downward (abdominal aspect) (See Plate 1). As the diaphragm contracts, it flattens, and pulls down towards the abdomen. This has the effect of decreasing the pressure in the thorax and increasing it in the abdomen. Negative thoracic pressure draws air in through the trachea into the lungs: when we breathe in, our lungs fill with air, and our abdomen normally protrudes. This is called abdominal breathing. It is also possible to increase the volume of the thorax by moving the ribs up and down. The ribs, which are hinged to the vertebrae, are connected to each other by smaller (intercostal) muscles. The rib cage is also connected to the collar-bone (clavicle) and the neck muscles. Using these muscles allows the ribs to move to a small degree. This type of breathing, thoracic breathing, is less effective, more effortful, and generally not used in proper vocal technique. A comparison of breathing techniques among actors revealed that the accomplished actor uses more abdominal breathing, and that this abdominal breathing shows greater variation and control than in his novice actor counterpart.

The abdomen also plays a significant role in voice production. During inhalation, as the diaphragm contracts and descends, the abdominal cavity is compressed and its contents protrude. The muscles of the abdominal wall relax to accommodate this compression. Exhalation during quiet breathing is passive, as the contracted diaphragm relaxes, and the abdominal contents expand to exert upward pressure. During singing and dramatic vocalization, however, exhalation is controlled and active: the muscles in the abdominal wall (the recti and the obliques) contract, pushing the abdominal contents up against the diaphragm. The effect is that of pushing in the plunger of a syringe: air is expelled at a controlled rate of flow through the glottis (laryngeal aperture). The muscles which act in concert then are: the diaphragm, contracting during inhalation, and the abdominals, during exhalation. It is worth emphasizing that the diaphragm is capable of only one active movement, which is contraction (descent). During exhalation and voice production the diaphragm does not contract, and is only a passive partition. Many singers are not aware of this fact, and fancifully attribute the act of breathing to other mechanisms. When asked about the breathing mechanism, one singer spoke about the passive descent of the diaphragm which resulted from air entering the lungs. Many singers image the act of inspiration as a passive event, 'allowing the air to enter', or 'letting the air fall into the lungs'. All of these images are physiologically incorrect.

When expiration occurs, the diaphragm is flaccid, and is passively pushed up by the contents of a contracting abdominal cavity. Supporting the voice from the diaphragm is therefore a concept with no anatomical basis. Support of the voice actually comes from the abdominal muscles, rather than the diaphragm. This in-and-out movement is most effective when the supporting structures do not move. These structures, the pelvis and the back, provide points of attachment for the muscles of respiration, and must be held immobile for optimal respiratory movements.

General muscle tone

The degree of muscular activity in parts of the body not directly involved in respiratory movements is also important. Tension in any muscle group heightens the tension in all other groups, leading to tightness, strain and less effective voice production. Tension in the neck, lower back or even the limbs heightens the tone in muscles directly involved in singing, increasing the effort and decreasing efficiency. Part of the singer's art is to develop conscious control of postures and movements which are normally reflexive, and exert that control in isolating muscles which must contract, muscles which must relax, and muscles which must be in a state of effortless tone.

Techniques such as Alexander and Feldenkrais are helpful in developing conscious awareness on posture and movement.

Phonation and singing

Vowel sounds are produced when the airstream is continuous; consonants by more or less complete interruption of the stream by interposition of various parts of the tongue, teeth and lips. Singing, for the most part, consists of long phrases and emphasizes vowels. Speech, particularly conversation rather than declamation, emphasizes consonants. The contrast is especially marked if, for example, Russian and German are considered rather than Italian and French – which is one of the reasons why the latter are easier to sing.

The larynx

As mentioned, the larynx is the sound generator on which most interest has been focused. The larynx evolved originally not as the organ of phonation, but as a sphincter which protects the lower airway during swallowing. The larynx is divided into three parts: the glottic part, referring to the true vocal folds; the subglottic part, referring to the area below the glottis; and the supraglottic part, referring to the structures above the vocal folds.

The main structures of the laryngeal framework are the thyroid cartilage and the cricoid cartilage. The thyroid cartilage of the larynx has a triangular shape. The two sides are formed of rigid cartilage and meet anteriorly to form a keel. The top of this keel, called the thyroid notch, can be seen and felt as the Adam's apple (See Plate 2). The two wings (alae) of the thyroid cartilage flare posterolaterally, and are open across the back. The thyroid cartilage rests on a rigid ring of cartilage, the cricoid cartilage. The thyroid cartilage hinges on the cricoid on both sides, and can swing up and down, much like the visor of a knight's helmet. Unlike the thyroid, the cricoid forms a complete and rigid ring around the upper end of the trachea. It is flattened posteriorly and rounded anteriorly, like a signet ring (See Plate 2).

The thyroid and cricoid cartilages constitute the main 'skeleton' of the larynx. The cricoid is attached to the first ring of the trachea by fibrous tissue which allows for both strength and some flexibility.

As already mentioned, the larynx's importance for survival rests in its function as a protective sphincter. Protection of lungs from saliva, food, liquid, and other ingested material is in fact so vital, that there is not one but three different sphincters within the larynx. The lowest, immediately above the cricoid, is formed by the true vocal folds (cords). These are thin slips of muscle and a ligament, covered by mucous membrane, which attach to the inside of the thyroid keel anteriorly (See Plate 3). Posteriorly, each vocal fold attaches to an arytenoid cartilage. The arytenoids are tiny jug-shaped cartilages which sit on either side on top of the flattened cricoid lamina (See Plate 2). They are controlled by fine muscles, which allow them to swivel apart or together, slide toward each other, and tip forward (See Plate 5). The airway between the vocal folds is called the glottis, or glottic aperture, and is like an isosceles triangle in cross section. Its equal sides are formed by the vocal folds, and its base by the muscle and soft tissue between the arytenoids. The apex of the triangle is formed by the anterior commissure where the vocal folds are attached to

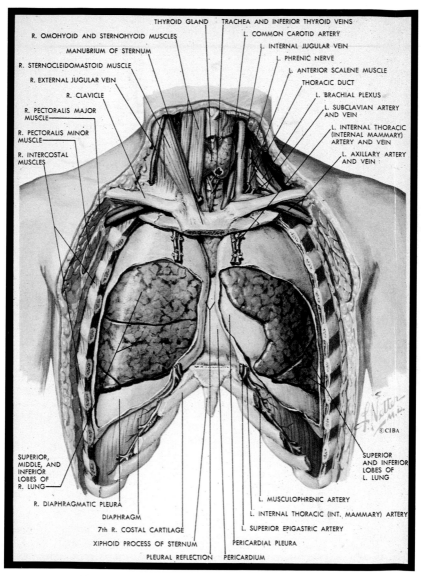

Plate 1 Thoracic cage: anterior relations

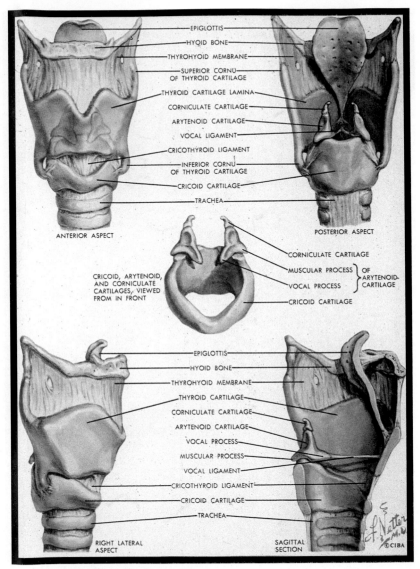

EPIGLOTTIS
HYOID BONE
THYROHYOID MEMBRANE
SUPERIOR CORNU OF THYROID CARTILAGE
THYROID CARTILAGE LAMINA
CORNICULATE CARTILAGE
ARYTENOID CARTILAGE
VOCAL LIGAMENT
CRICOTHYROID LIGAMENT
INFERIOR CORNU OF THYROID CARTILAGE
CRICOID CARTILAGE
TRACHEA

ANTERIOR ASPECT

POSTERIOR ASPECT

CRICOID, ARYTENOID, AND CORNICULATE CARTILAGES, VIEWED FROM IN FRONT

CORNICULATE CARTILAGE
MUSCULAR PROCESS } OF ARYTENOID CARTILAGE
VOCAL PROCESS
CRICOID CARTILAGE

EPIGLOTTIS
HYOID BONE
THYROHYOID MEMBRANE
THYROID CARTILAGE
CORNICULATE CARTILAGE
ARYTENOID CARTILAGE
VOCAL PROCESS
MUSCULAR PROCESS
VOCAL LIGAMENT
CRICOTHYROID LIGAMENT
CRICOID CARTILAGE
TRACHEA

RIGHT LATERAL ASPECT

SAGITTAL SECTION

© CIBA

Plate 2 Cartilages of larynx

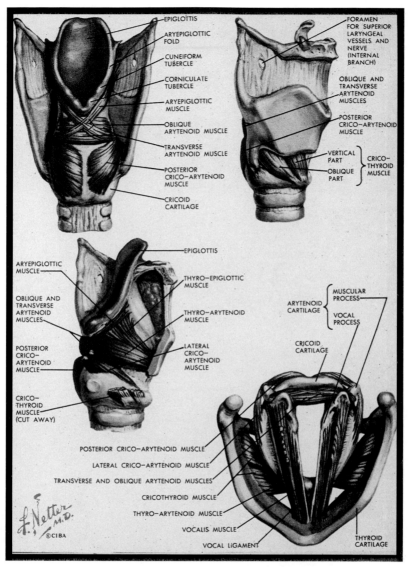

Plate 3 Intrinsic muscles of larynx

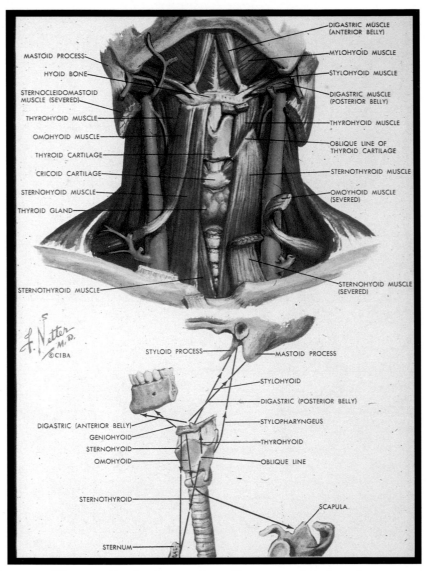

Plate 4 Extrinsic muscles of larynx and their action

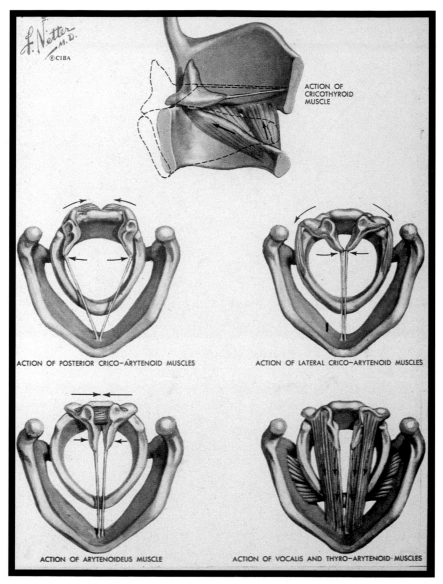

Plate 5 Action of intrinsic muscles of larynx

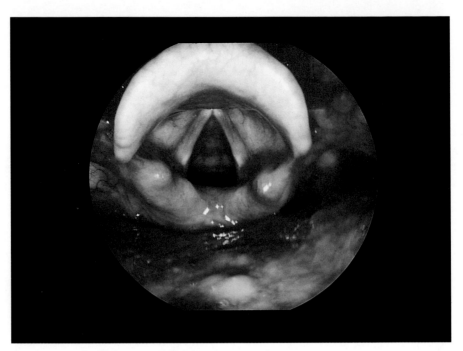

Plate 6 Normal larynx

the inner surface of the thyroid cartilage. When the arytenoids swivel or pull apart (abduction), the base of the triangle widens, and the airway opens. When the arytenoids come together (adduction), the base of the triangle narrows. When the arytenoids (and the attached vocal folds) are progressively adducted, the airway narrows to a slit, and becomes completely closed. It is in this adducted position that phonation occurs, and this will be discussed at length later (See Plate 5).

Above each vocal fold is a broader fold of mucous membrane, the false vocal fold (cord). As the name implies, the false vocal folds look a bit like the true folds, but are not normally 'vocal', i.e. involved in phonation. The false folds are not only attached to the arytenoids, but also contain some muscle, which allows them to contract. They lack the fine control of the true folds, but can be squeezed together, along with the true folds, to protect the airway. They thus form the second set of sphincters which protects the lungs. The false and true vocal folds in cross-section look like shelves which project in towards the centre of the airway. They are separated by a small pouch, or pocket, called the laryngeal ventricle. The ventricle, and especially its anterior recess (saccule) is lined with mucus-producing glands which lubricate the vocal folds. In humans, this ventricle has no role in phonation, although in some lower animals (like frogs, apes and monkeys) it can be inflated and act as a resonator or additional air source during phonation.

The third, and highest, laryngeal sphincter is formed by the epiglottis (See Plates 2 and 3). This floppy, petal-shaped cartilage is attached at its base to the inner surface of the thyroid cartilage. The rounded petal portion projects up toward the base of the tongue. Its sides are connected by mucous membrane and some muscle fibres to the tips of the arytenoids behind and below it. These folds (aryepiglottic folds), along with the epiglottis in front and the arytenoids in the back encircle the airway. During swallowing, the epiglottis tips back, like the lid of a box; the aryepiglottic folds and arytenoids pull toward the centre of the airway, and together they close off the top of the larynx. By this mechanism, not only is the airway protected, but channels open up on either side of the epiglottis which allow the swallowed material to flow around the larynx posteriorly, and arrive behind the cricoid, at the upper end of the food passage (oesophagus). This constitutes the third, or supraglottic, sphincter.

Of equal importance to the protective action of these sphincters during swallowing is the powerful upward sliding movement of the entire larynx and attached trachea. This upward motion tucks the larynx close behind the base of the tongue, and under the epiglottis. A set of muscles, which suspend the larynx from the hyoid bone and the jaw allow this elevation to take place (See Plate 4). After swallowing, the larynx moves back down to its resting position in the neck. In keeping with the overriding importance of airway protection, the muscles which pull the larynx down (depressors) are not as powerful as those which raise it (elevators). This is somewhat analogous to the powerful muscles which close a crocodile's jaw, versus the weaker ones which open it. The significance of this fact becomes apparent to singers and actors who are untrained, or performers vocalizing with a great deal of muscular tension. Since laryngeal elevators overpower laryngeal depressors, these singers will often sing with a high larynx. Both externally and internally, the characteristic laryngeal posture caused by excessive muscle tension will reflect the domination of stronger muscles over weaker ones.

The larynx thus far has been described as a sphincter. It protects the lower airway during swallowing by elevating toward the back of the tongue, and closing, bringing together the triple valves of the true folds, the false folds and the supraglottic structures. How does this guardian of the lower airway produce voice? The larynx, as already mentioned, is an organ which can open or close. With the vocal folds (glottis) in the open position (Plate 6), it allows the free flow of air to the lungs during respiration. In the closed position, it protects the airway, and allows the diversion of ingested food and liquid posteriorly, into the oesophagus. This closure is usually instantaneous, reflexive and momentary, coinciding with swallowing. It is also possible to close the larynx voluntarily. In this situation, the vocal folds are forcibly held together, and air pressure in the lower airway is increased by pushing the abdominal contents and the diaphragm up. This pushing against a closed glottis (the Valsalva manoeuvre) facilitates certain actions, such as lifting and straining.

The subglottic air pressure can be increased as long as the vocal folds are held together. Once the air pressure is greater than the force adducting the folds, the folds will be pushed apart, and air will flow through the larynx. Phonation (and singing) consists of balancing the adductive force on the vocal folds, and the sub-glottic air pressure. These are balanced so closely, that as air pushes the vocal folds apart, decreasing subglottic pressure, the vocal folds immediately return to the closed position. Air pressure again builds up until the folds are blown apart. This repeated process results in tiny puffs of air which set the vocal folds vibrating. The folds are not like stiff reeds, but rather like a trumpeter's lips, which are held under some muscular tension, but open and close rapidly, creating a buzzing sound. In this way, the voice is formed. The frequency of the vocal fold vibration determines the pitch of the sound.

This phenomenon is similar for speech, singing, and other vocal utterances. The main difference lies in the fact that singing in-volves a more prolonged and sustained voice production, while speech is usually a series of transient sounds.

The normal pitch range of vocalization means that the vocal folds must vibrate hundreds of times per second. They are uniquely suited for this extremely rapid and fine movement by their layered structure. The substance, or body, of the vocal fold consists of the thyroarytenoid (vocalis) muscle, which stretches between the arytenoid cartilage posteriorly and the inner surface of the thyroid cartilage anteriorly. This muscle can actively contract and relax, and can be also stretched passively by muscles which move the cartilages to which it is attached (cricothyroid and cricoarytenoid muscles) (See Plate 3). The vocalis muscle is rather bulky, and certainly not capable of rapid and minute oscillations. However, the cover of the vocal fold, consisting of a thin layer of mucous membrane, is. This is possible due to the loose and slippery attachment of this covering membrane to the underlying vocal ligament and muscle. This loose attachment, consisting of a gelatinous microlayer (Reinke's space), allows the mucous membrane to slide freely in response to air flow, while the vocalis muscle is held in position. The rapid and regular volley of air puffs (up to over 1000 times a second), creates a wave-like to-and-fro rolling of the mucosal cover: the folds are blown apart, slide back together, and are blown apart once more. The coming together of the edges is the result of two forces: once air has escaped through the glottis, the subglottic air pressure is tempor-arily decreased, and the approximating muscular forces of the larynx are temporarily dominant. The rapid flow of air between the edges itself creates a force (Venturi effect) which pulls the free edges towards each other. Once the glottis is closed, subglottic air pressure again builds up, and the cycle repeats. Although this takes place much faster than the eye can discern, it can be visualized by high-speed photography, or by stroboscopy.

Muscular control of vocal fold tension is complex, and involves several muscle groups acting in fine coordination. These muscles are classified as extrinsic and intrinsic. Extrinsic muscles (See Plate 4) connect the larynx to adjacent supporting structures such as the hyoid bone and sternum, whereas intrinsic muscles (See Plate 5) connect one part of the larynx to another. Different groups of muscles are used in producing the full vocal range. The lower part of the soprano voice, called chest register, is determined primarily by tension in the vocalis and arytenoid muscles. The upper part, or head voice, is controlled by the cricothyroid muscle, which tilts the thyroid cartilage forward, stretching and thinning the lips of the vocal folds. The transition from one mode of muscle activity to the other (chest to head voice) is awkward, and must be smoothly executed. This 'break', called the passaggio, usually occurs at E–F above middle C. The smooth and effortless transition through the passaggio without loss of range, resonance or flexibility must be learned, and is the hallmark of technical mastery. The natural break in the voice which reflects a change in muscle activity is sometimes accentuated for effect, such as seen with yodelling.

Paradoxically, the phonatory movements of the larynx are exactly opposite to its protective actions. For good singing, the larynx must be lowered, not raised, and the supraglottic areas kept open, approximating only the true vocal folds. Rather than squeezing the vocal folds together in a reflexive 'all-or-nothing' fashion, the singer must bring them together with a high degree of sensitivity and control, balancing the approximation against the pressure of the air being pushed out from the lungs. From the laryngeal point of view, good singing is a rather unnatural function!

The supraglottic larynx and pharynx

So far, we have examined the power source (lungs) and sound generator (larynx) involved in the voice. In many ways, however, the most important component of voice formation lies in the structures above the larynx.

When the newly-formed voice leaves the vocal folds, it has a raw, bleating sound. It is reminiscent of the sound generated by blowing a jet of air across a rotating perforated paper disc. It is unpleasant, and certainly not musical. Voice owes its true quality (projection, colour, expressiveness) to the supraglottic compartments of the vocal tract. These include the parts of the larynx above the vocal folds, the various parts of the pharynx and the mouth. (Contrary to popular assumption, the nose and sinuses contribute little in this regard.)

The supraglottic part of the larynx includes cavities defined by the false vocal folds, ventricles, aryepiglottic folds and the epiglottis. Above these is the pharynx, divided into three parts: the part directly continuous with the back of the mouth (oropharynx); the part above this, and behind the palate and the nose (nasopharynx); and the part between the oropharynx and the larynx (hypopharynx).

These supraglottic spaces are divided into compartments by folds which act as walls and baffles, including the soft palate and the epiglottis. Although the raw voice leaving the vocal folds is a buzzing, unfocused sound, its frequency can be controlled by the rate of air flow, and the sound typically contains many frequencies, some louder than others. It is the function of the supraglottic compartments to purify this sound and this occurs because these compartments function as resonators.

Every air-containing cavity is a potential resonator. This means that the air volume within will preferentially vibrate at certain frequencies. The resonant frequency of such cavities depends on the ratio between its physical dimensions, and the length of the sound wave which is transmitted to it. When the wavelength of sound and the space form is in a simple mathematical ratio, the air contained will vibrate, and the cavity will resonate. Resonance has the effect of amplifying certain frequencies, in effect magnifying them above the loudness of other frequencies contained in the original sound. The buzzing, impure laryngeal utterance passes through these supraglottic compartments, and becomes purified and strengthened.

If these cavities were rigid-walled boxes, only certain frequencies could be easily amplified, much like a valveless bugle.

However, the walls of the supraglottic resonators are mobile. The larynx above the vocal folds (i.e. the aryepiglottic folds, the epiglottis, the false folds and the ventricles) may be opened or closed. Similarly, the hypopharynx may be changed in shape and size by lowering the larynx, constricting or opening the side walls of the pharynx (pyriform fossae), and moving the tongue. Likewise, the shape of the mouth is highly adjustable. The effect is more like playing a trombone: adjusting the length of the slide allows the player to sound the full scale of tones. The singer, by manipulating the size, shape and position of the supralaryngeal compartments, can select, shape, colour and amplify a vast vocal range. Using the various laryngeal muscles and varying the supraglottic resonators, the human voice has a total range of five octaves, from two and a half octaves below middle C to two and a half octaves above. Of course the predominant range of an individual's voice is predetermined by the anatomy of the vocal mechanism. A bass cannot sing in the tenor range, and most sopranos cannot sing alto.

Nose, mouth, tongue and palate

Once sound has risen from the back of the throat, it passes through the upper resonators, which include the nasopharynx, nasal cavity and mouth. The sinuses are often thought of as important resonators, but their actual effect on the voice is not clear. Singers who have undergone sinus surgery do not usually experience a change in the voice, although their perception of where the sound is felt may be altered. Similarly, nasal resonance is more a proprioceptive than an acoustic reality. Punt has stated that a singer with a nose full of polyps will sound not significantly worse than one with open nasal passages, although he may pay a price in terms of dry mouth, impaired respiration and altered physical perception of vibration.

The sound is further shaped by the mouth. The most mobile portion of the mouth, the tongue, greatly affects the acoustic properties of this cavity, and singers therefore learn to flatten the tongue and maximize the volume of the oral cavity. Elevating the palate has a similar effect, and this motion further funnels the sounds through the mouth and minimizes nasal air leakage. A mobile and finely controlled palate is essential. Any impediment to palate elevation, such as massively enlarged tonsils, or scarring of the tonsil pillars following improperly performed tonsillectomy, may present a problem in this regard. Articulation is for the most part due to the action of the lips, tongue tip and teeth. Laryngeal articulation (coupe glottique) may on occasion be used for special effect, but is in the long run deleterious, and is therefore to be avoided.

Acoustic parameters of the voice

Although voice quality is a complex phenomenon which for the most part is in the ear of the beholder, certain physical parameters are inherent in all voice production, and should be understood.

Sound intensity is the chief determinant of voice loudness. Intensity is determined in part by the amplitude of vocal fold vibrations and this depends primarily on breath pressure. The size, shape and position of the resonators also play an important role in intensity. Even the loudest voice, however would be easily covered by an orchestra, were it not for a special quality, referred to as the 'ring' of the operatic voice. This has been shown to correspond to an overtone, in the region of 2800–3400 Hz, which is probably generated immediately above the vocal folds

Pitch depends on frequency of vocal fold vibration which mainly depends on: length, thickness, breadth and stiffness of the vibrating part of the vocal folds; muscle forces tending to close the glottis (appose the folds); and breath pressure. The increase in breath pressure tends to raise pitch, a phenomenon which is usually easily corrected by adjusting vocal fold pressure. When the singer must perform on swollen folds, there is a tendency to push with the unintended result that the pitch may be sharp.

Quality (timbre) is defined by the relative emphasis of harmonic partials (overtones) which depends on selective amplification of overtones inherent in the laryngeal sound by the particular shape, dimensions and consistency of walls of the series of resonators (especially pharynx and mouth). Patients with inflammation of the pharynx will experience a change in voice quality, since the pharyngeal walls are oedematous, and the supporting muscles inflamed. Patients with vocal nodules may be able to produce a double tone (diplophonia), because as the swellings approximate each other, they define two separate and freely vibrating segments, on either side of the nodules. This phenomenon is analogous to the harmonics created by a partially stopped string on the violin.

The voice produced by the singer is constantly monitored in two ways: by audition and by proprioception. Certainly, the singer hears the voice produced, and hears it in two ways: sound leaving the mouth is picked up by the ears (air conduction), but sound in the throat is also directly transmitted to the inner ears through the tissues of the throat, neck and bony skeleton (bone conduction). In addition, the physical vibration of the tissues is sensed by nerve endings, which create a physical (non-auditory) sensation. This mechanism, called proprioception, is felt maximally in different parts of the vocal tract, depending on how the voice is produced. It is proprioception which gives rise to expressions such as 'singing in the mask'. Singers can physically 'locate' the sound anywhere, from the breastbone through the top of the head using proprioception.

In summary, the act of singing is a highly complex simultaneous and constantly varying set of neuromuscular actions. The voice is powered by the lungs. Exhalation is minutely counterbalanced by constriction of the vocal folds which generates tones of different frequencies. The laryngeal sound is shaped by the pharynx, palate and mouth, giving it purity, shape and projection. The sound produced is constantly monitored, and adjusted according to perceived variation between what is generated and what is demanded by the singer's musical intelligence.

The various individual parts of the vocal mechanism act in concert, and, for the most part, in an unconscious and reflexive fashion. One of the voice professional's tasks is to develop conscious awareness and purposeful control over these actions. For example, lifting the palate, flattening the tongue and lowering the larynx are manoeuvres which the untrained student cannot reliably achieve. None the less, no voice professional, regardless of expertise, can achieve individual conscious control over every muscle in the larynx. Excessive anatomical analysis, at the expense of a more holistic approach may be counterproductive. The ideal approach requires a practical understanding of anatomy and physiology, guided by an aesthetic and musical consciousness.

Development of the larynx and the voice

Anatomical and physiological changes in the larynx begin before birth, and continue throughout life. At birth, the thyroid and hyoid are cartilaginous, and are attached to each other. Thereafter, they separate and the slow process of ossification (cartilage turning to bone) begins. By the age of 2 years, the hyoid bone has begun to ossify. The thyroid and cricoid cartilages start to ossify during the early 20s. The arytenoid cartilages ossify later in the 30s. By the age of 65 virtually the entire laryngeal skeleton is normally ossified. This process involves the thyroid, cricoid and arytenoid, which are made of hyaline cartilage. However, the epiglottis and tiny accessory cartilages are made of elastic, rather than hyaline, cartilage, and remain soft.

In general, the onset of ossification occurs later and is less extensive in women and the entire process is variable. This process of ossification is part of maturation, and does not normally affect the voice.

The epiglottis in a very young child is omega-shaped and thickened and it does not adopt its normal adult outline until puberty. At birth, there are only minor differences between the male and female larynx. The differences are negligible until puberty, when rapid growth of the male larynx leads to dramatic differences between the sexes. The larynx at birth is high in the neck, resting at the level of the third and fourth cervical vertebrae, but it descends to the level of the sixth vertebrae by the age of 5. The gradual descent of the larynx continues so that between the ages of 15 and 20 the larynx lies at the level of the seventh cervical vertebra. Throughout life the larynx continues to descend and consequently the vocal tract length relationships change and the voice tends to become lower. The membranous vibrating portion of the vocal fold of the infant is the same length as the cartilaginous or non-vibrating part, but by adulthood the membranous portion becomes approximately two thirds of the vocal fold length.

Whereas the vocal fold length in an infant is only 6–8 mm, this increases to 12–17 mm in the adult female and to 17–23 mm in the adult male. There is a corresponding growth in other aspects of the larynx during this period. The unmodulated fundamental frequency of the larynx at birth is around 500 Hz (about one octave above middle C). As the child develops, the predominant pitch of the speaking voice (mean fundamental frequency) drops, thus, the frequency at 8 years is approximately 275 Hz. Until puberty, male and female larynges are about the same size and during childhood the highest and lowest sounds a child can produce (the physiological frequency range), remain rather constant. With maturation, however, the child is able to produce musically acceptable sounds throughout an increasing percentage of his frequency range. Sataloff points out that between the ages of 6 and 16 the important developmental changes are not in absolute range (which remains constant at about two and a half octaves), but rather improved efficiency, control and quality. Recognition of this principle is essential in training young voices. The aim should be to strengthen and take advantage of the natural developmental process rather than concentrating too early and too much on exercises that are designed to increase the extremes of range. Damage may ensue if young, fragile voices are frequently stretched to and beyond their limits.

Pubertal changes

Puberty, with its associated rapid growth, brings about significant changes in the voice. The voice typically deepens, and grows more resonant. While these changes are the result of several factors (increased respiratory capacity, greater muscle mass, lower laryngeal position), they relate most importantly to anatomical and physiological changes within the larynx itself.

The age of onset of puberty varies greatly, and is determined by factors such as race, heredity and perhaps general nutrition. Puberty tends to come later in the colder northern hemisphere than in warmer climates and generally occurs at an earlier age than was the case 50 years ago. In North America, puberty generally begins between 8 and 15 years for females and between $9\frac{1}{2}$ and 14 for males. The process is usually complete in girls between the ages of 12 and $16\frac{1}{2}$ and in boys approximately between $13\frac{1}{2}$ and 18 years.

The voice changes during puberty are caused by rapid and significant alterations in the anatomy of the larynx that occur simultaneously with the development of other secondary sex characteristics. Female vocal folds grow 1–3.5 mm whereas male vocal folds grow 4–6 mm in length. The thyroid cartilage angle (Adam's apple) of the male becomes more acute (about 90°), so that the adolescent male larynx becomes more prominent. This prominence is also accentuated by the descent of the larynx in the neck. The thyroid cartilage angle of the female, however, remains at about 120°, and the larynx remains relatively smaller and higher, leaving the Adam's apple less prominent.

The fundamental pitch of the voice changes, and becomes temporarily unstable, fluctuating unpredictably (and uncontrollably) between the high pitch of childhood and low pitch (often an octave lower) of adulthood. This yodelling is referred to as mutation, or mutational falsetto. During puberty the male voice drops significantly, averaging a fundamental frequency of about 130 Hz at 18 years, whereas the female voice drops less, and averages roughly 220–225 Hz when the voice change is complete. Voice mutation is generally complete in both sexes by the age of 15 years, although in some males a mutational falsetto persists into adulthood, resulting in a yodelling type voice (puberphonia).

At the completion of puberty, the lower limit of the male voice has descended on average by an octave, while the upper limit had dropped by a sixth. No certain conclusions can be reached from a boy's voice about the quality and type of voice that he will develop as an adult. A child soprano voice often becomes a baritone or a basso, while altos frequently develop into tenors. Caruso sang alto in a church choir.

Other laryngeal changes are common to both sexes. The epiglottis increases in size, elongates and flattens and the laryngeal mucosa becomes thicker and stronger. The bulk of the lymphoid tissue in the pharynx and nasopharynx, i.e. tonsillar and adenoidal tissue, markedly decreases in size, and the neck itself elongates.

These supraglottic changes affect the resonance, harmonic spectrum and projection of the voice. The chest expands, increasing vital capacity, and the power of the voice. There is usually a greater thoracic enlargement in the male with a resulting greater vital capacity of the lungs.

Vocal training and the young larynx

The tessitura of the child's voice is higher than that of the adult because the larynx is smaller. The volume is less because the bellows are less powerful, and the quality is thinner, because the supraglottic resonators are smaller.

Children have constantly changing voices with very delicate muscles and fragile mucosa. They are particularly vulnerable to abusive vocal habits and especially the demands of prolonged 'belting' and the prolonged mimicking of their rock star idols. Children often begin their musical careers singing Broadway or West End musicals in summer camp productions, or trying to emulate the amplified and electronically enhanced voices they hear on the radio, both with potentially disastrous consequences.

Parents of children who want to sing are sometimes told that the child is 'too young' for voice lessons, and should just be allowed to 'sing naturally'. This is bad advice: provided the young performer has a caring and knowledgeable teacher, it is reasonable to start the young singer on training as soon as a distinct enthusiasm is shown. Parents should distinguish between voice teachers and vocal coaches. A child needs a teacher to learn the craft of singing, rather than a coach who works on a specific performance.

Initial training may be nothing more than instruction on breathing and avoiding injurious practice. Bad technical advice and the pushing of a young voice rather than slow and gradual gentle nurturing may result in vocal problems throughout a career by improper development of the muscles of singing. Once improper vocal usage has developed, either through neglect or premature pushing, it may be doubly difficult to erase bad habits and imprint good ones. A taxing performance for a child in a demanding musical on stage can, if continued night after night, result in vocal abuse causing pathological changes. This is particularly so in musicals where a shouted or belted quality is sought

(Annie, Oliver, etc.). Even if the production is amplified, reducing the need for projection, the technique needed to produce this quality of voice is potentially harmful. It is far wiser therefore, for the producer to have several child leads who alternate their appearances rather then precipitating vocal injury in one individual.

Although classical musicians are more aware of the limitations of children's voices, misguided zeal can lead to problems even in this repertoire. The enthusiasm of a choir master to encourage a boy soprano or alto to maintain his treble voice at the onset of puberty can be hazardous.

Serious vocal studies should not begin in boys before the age of 18–19 and girls before 17 years, but the young singer's true voice type may not be manifest for several years. Young men who have sung tenor parts in a choir may in fact be baritones. Such classifications in any case should only be regarded as a guide and are artificial. Really deep bassos – the basso profundo of the Italians – and the high tenors and true contraltos are very rare. The majority of voices are found in the middle ranges. However, a heavy premium of having glory and money is placed on having very high or very low voices and the temptation to extend the natural range is great. Many baritones have ruined their voices by masquerading as tenors and many mezzosopranos invaded the soprano territory to discover, too late, that one cannot flout nature with impunity. Some of the most famous contraltos have actually been mezzosopranos and the early deterioration of their voices is a sad commentary on overextension of the range. The dramatic and the lyric voices represent different types in both voice and different personalities of the singer.

The selection of the first teacher for a young singer is of paramount importance. The great artist is often a poor teacher who forces his or her own technique on the students. Many great artists have great natural aptitude and have not encountered technical problems such as their students may face. Such a performer may lack pedagogic versatility, and the ability to put vital information into words. Some of the best teachers have not had great performing careers themselves.

Students should also beware of teachers who only take on already accomplished pupils. A good teacher is successful with many students of differing abilities. It is important that the serious young singer avoid smoking, and limit alcohol consumption to a minimum. He should work on the control of the voice in the middle register, avoid testing the high tones, and avoid giving public performances until 19 or 20 years of age. There is obviously a variation, for sometimes a student may reach adequate proficiency by the age of 18, while others may not have reasonable maturity until 21 to 22. The voice is growing and the knowledge of how to control it should also increase.

A singer must be taught to use the best voice type (soprano, tenor, etc), if not, voice problems may emerge at a later date. The high tones which come effortlessly and without practice should be the extreme extent of the register, and should define the singer's voice type. With some singers an incorrect classification of voice type may not become evident for years. The first problem usually arises when they are maintaining high notes, and they experience difficulty in changing registers (i.e. the passagio).

Young singers often attempt to sound older than their vocal years, which is a dangerous tendency and is not an infrequent cause of vocal dysfunction. A beautiful voice which is small and light should be nurtured gradually, and not broken in on heavy dramatic roles. The majority of commercially marketed pop voices are artificial creations of the amplifier that would sound tiny and shaky if the singer ever tried to sing without clutching a microphone.

Even with gentle nurture, each voice has certain strengths and limitations inherent in its anatomy. It is the task of the teacher to discover and develop these attributes, and nowhere is this more important than in the young singer at the beginning of his or her studies.

3

Age and voice

Normal ageing of the larynx

Ageing is a gradual and lifelong process which brings about structural and functional changes in the larynx. Along with the effects of ageing, the mature voice also reflects compensatory vocal strategies which have been adopted, either consciously or unconsciously, by the vocal artist.

With ageing, the voice typically loses power and resonance. There are also characteristic changes in pitch, which are more noticeable in males than in females. The mean fundamental frequency drops steadily in females from 225 Hz in the 20 to 30-year-old age group to about 195 Hz in the 80 to 90-year-old age group. In males however, the fundamental frequency of the speaking voice drops until roughly the fifth decade, after which it gradually rises because of the decreased bulk and elasticity of the vocal folds. The terms used to describe vocal quality changes resulting from this rise include 'thin', 'reedy' and 'breathy'. Pitch change is not so noticeable among females.

In the male, attempts at compensation for pitch changes can result in a gravelly and 'vocal fry' type of phonation, with easy fatiguing of the voice and consequent increased vocal effort. The audible breathiness and fry correlates with apparent shortening and bowing of the true folds on indirect laryngoscopy (Plate 7). Less bowing may be noted if vocal fold lengthening can be achieved by higher-pitched phonation and the voice may become considerably less dysphonic when the patient is encouraged to speak at a higher pitch. With ageing, there is generally a loss of muscle mass, suppleness, and muscular fine control. In some cases, this deterioration in fine control is worsened by tremor, which may be essential, or related to degenerative changes in the brain (Parkinsonism, cerebellar disease). In addition, patients with joint diseases (particularly rheumatoid arthritis) may occasionally also develop stiffening of the laryngeal joints with a consequent decrease in the range of movement of the laryngeal cartilages.

As female singers reach the menopause, oestrogen lack causes obvious changes in the muscles and mucosa of the vocal tract. The same drying, thinning and atrophy that is seen in the mouth, eyes and genital tract may affect the larynx. Changes that appear in the voice can be counteracted for many years with hormone replacement therapy (HRT), as discussed elsewhere. The most physiological way of dealing with this is to give a mixture of oestrogens and progesterone. The dose should be monitored by blood hormone levels. Occasionally an oestrogen/androgen combination is prescribed by endocrinologists for dysmenorrhoea or contraception in women. Pure androgens may be given for treatment of breast cancer. These male hormones cause a lowered pitch and impart a darker colour to the voice. It is important that the female singer is aware of the irreversible ill effects of androgens on the voice.

The general lack of muscle tone which tends to occur with the ageing process can be largely avoided or even reversed by general fitness exercises. Press ups, weight lifting and jogging should be avoided, but rapid walking, swimming and aerobics are entirely suitable. Although these exercises do not train the laryngeal muscles specifically, there are benefits from increased muscle tone of the neck, back, thorax and abdomen. Furthermore, exercising improves circulation to every organ, including the brain and the vocal tract. In the older age group the lungs lose their elasticity, the thoracic cage grows more rigid and the abdominal muscle mass tends to deteriorate. A singer whose general condition does not allow him to hurry up a few flights of stairs without becoming short of breath is unlikely to be able to sustain good abdominal support throughout a taxing concert, recital or opera. When the power source of the voice is decreased, compensatory and excessive use of the neck and tongue muscles ensues, with resulting vocal dysfunction. A regimen of gradual conditioning exercises under an experienced sports instructor or trainer will not only improve general muscle tone and function, but also restore the feeling of 'well-being'.Vocal exercises with an experienced teacher, which emphasize agility, flexibility and support go a long way toward delaying the deleterious effects of ageing.

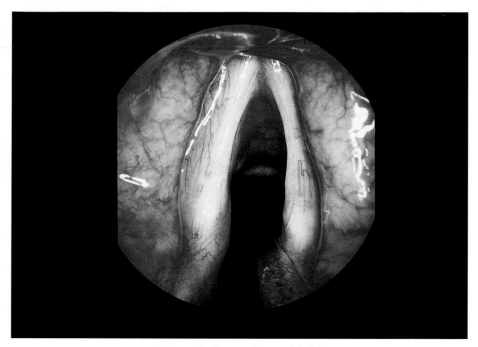

Plate 7 Bowed vocal folds

Acoustic instability has also been associated with advancing age, particularly in females. These minute variations of voice pitch and loudness, manifested by shimmer and jitter, appear to correlate more with physiological rather than chronological age, occurring more often in elderly subjects in poor general health. Breathiness may result from either impaired breath support or incomplete glottic closure, secondary to bowing of the vocal folds or decreased mobility of the cricoarytenoid joints. Bowing and atrophy of the vocal folds is seen in a large number of elderly individuals, whereas in the 40-year age group this is unusual. These gross changes correlate with microscopic findings showing degeneration of the laryngeal muscles and increased fragmentation of elastic fibres in the submucosa. There are also alterations in neuromuscular control. Decreased efficiency of the sensory/motor reflexes (e.g. gag reflex) has been substantiated by finding a reduced number of nerve endings in the elderly larynx. The mucous membrane of the senescent vocal folds are thinned and atrophic. Impaired lubrication of the folds is likely to be the result of atrophy and decrease in the number of mucous glands in the larynx.

There are many other causes for vocal changes in the elderly and these include depression, muscle tension dysphonia, the use of drying medications and the voice changes associated with smoking and drinking. Functional dysphonia in the elderly may also result from misguided attempts to compensate for the effects of ageing. For example, males may attempt to maintain a lower pitch, whereas females try to elevate their pitch. Inadequate breath support may result in excessively harsh glottic closure. Patients with a hearing loss or even those who attempt to communicate on a frequent basis with other hearing impaired elderly friends or relatives may develop functional dysphonia.

While the rate of ageing is to some degree genetically predetermined, its effects can be accelerated by injudicious singing. The scoop, the wide, wobbly and uncentred vibrato and the loss of accurate pitch in women may reflect either age, voice abuse or, most commonly, both.

The ageing person tends to lose teeth. Partial loss of dentition can alter the articulation. The edentulous patient sometimes has ill-fitting dentures which slip to such a degree that they produce articulatory errors. Loss of dentition may cause problems with occlusion, articulation and pain in the temporomandibular joint. It is sometimes wise to have an impression made while dentition is normal so that if problems arise at a later date, dentures can be fashioned similar to the person's natural teeth. Osteointegrated dental implants should be seriously considered for they are more satisfactory all round. Older patients and especially edentulous patients, also tend to complain of a dry mouth, due to the diminution of the amount of saliva secreted. However, many of these problems can be reduced by meticulous oral hygiene, maintaining a high fluid intake and on occasions using artificial saliva.

In the general management of a performer, it is important that a voice professional in his 60s does not undertake the same taxing roles that he took in his stride in his 40s. He may wish to accept more lyric rather than dramatic roles and, in planning a tour, must allow time for increased rest and recovery between commitments. The autumn of a career is also a time to consider shorter works rather than operas, and to weigh the advantages of 'crossing over' to a less demanding popular repertoire.

However, with awareness of these limitations and due diligence in maintaining general physical health, the singer will enjoy very many rewarding and fulfilling extra years of performances given to enthusiastic and appreciative audiences.

The wise artist, if financial considerations permit, will prefer to end her professional career with dignity, albeit sorrowfully, rather than continue a losing fight until all beauty has left her once admired tones. Intelligent operatic singers, in the autumn of their career, will limit their appearances to non-taxing operas and emphasize lieder, oratorios and popular songs which are shorter and can be more carefully chosen to emphasize the beauty remaining to the voice.

Attributes of a good
vocal performer

A great deal has been written on the natural attributes of a good singer. It is clear that two singers, both of similar quality may have travelled very different paths to arrive at the same level of performance. One singer may have a 'natural talent', with a capacious and flexible vocal instrument, and innate abilities of musical kinaesthetics and mimicry. The other may have had to put in arduous years of vocal apprenticeship, classes on movement and diction, and possibly numerous sessions of psychotherapy. The end result for the listener may be similar, but there is a great difference in the two singers' aptitudes.

Physical attributes conducive to good singing which have been cited include high and broad cheekbones, a large and wide mouth, a capacious pharynx and strong vocal folds. The actual appearance of the vocal folds may give some indication of where the singer's range should naturally lie, although this appearance may at times be deceptive. As a broad generalization, soprano vocal folds are usually white or even bluish-white and narrow, while a basso has broad and substantial folds which may always be slightly pink, rather than white. A large thoracic cage with ample lung capacity, strong and flexible trunk and limbs may be beneficial. Chronic respiratory illness, such as asthma or allergy problems may be limiting, and should be rigorously treated.

An often debated issue pertains to body habitus. It has been suggested that a certain amount of weight is necessary to 'support' the voice. This may be a fallacy which arose from the historic fact that, at the turn of the century, many singers were shorter and stockier. Some of today's finest singers carry a great deal of weight but, equally, some of the best voices are produced by singers who are lean and agile. In general, we feel that a singer should be at his or her natural weight. While specific roles will require dieting, a singer who is significantly undernourished will have difficulty with stamina and vocal support.

On the other hand, careless eating habits which lead to frank obesity should also be controlled, since excessive weight strains the heart, and can sap energy which ought to be directed to the vocal apparatus.

Unfortunately, today's world of opera and musicals places greater emphasis on the visual appearance than in earlier days. Television cameras scrutinize the performer's face, body and acting attributes at close-up range. A wooden tenor who stands centre stage and sings is no more convincing than an obese Violetta ostensibly dying of consumption.

In terms of non-physical attributes, intelligence, both musical and general, is important. An opera singer must not only consistently produce a beautiful voice, but must be comfortable in three or four languages. She must be able to memorize a four act opera lasting several hours, and this memorization includes minutiae of staging, acting, elocution, as well as comic and tragic interaction with other cast members. She must be ready for any last-minute change or mishap on stage, and be able to carry off the whole process convincingly and with enough force to involve emotionally an audience of several thousand.

While a singer and actor will achieve success by maximizing their natural abilities, it is equally important to recognize the limitations of each vocal instrument. A common phenomenon among opera singers today is to push young voices, or smaller voices into heavier roles. In some cases this is premature, while in others it should never be done. Dire consequences will be suffered by the lyric soprano who in her early twenties attempts the heavier Verdi repertoire. It is unfortunate that today there is no longer a viable career for the fine smaller voice. Most classical singers feel they must make their impact in opera, and lieder and oratorios are no longer considered a full-time career alternative. Even if the voice is operatic in size and quality, singers must guard against the temptation (usually based on ambition, money or vanity) to sing beyond their tessitura. An equally treacherous path leads to stereotyping. A great bass-baritone who sings only Wagner will burn out sooner than one who also sings Mozart and Verdi, as well as lieder and oratorios. Crossing over to the popular repertoire, music that is usually less demanding, is also a viable alternative for the smaller voice, since amplification displays the beauty and musicality without the physical demands of the unamplified operatic stage.

Psychological aptitude is infrequently discussed, but vitally important. A performer must have a good sense of self, a confidence which projects beyond any feeling of insecurity. This appearance of confidence shows in the performer's carriage and in his interaction with colleagues and the public on and off stage. The eccentric primadonna of former times is less tolerated now, when the artist lives almost 24 hours a day in the public eye. A fickle and undependable temperament will soon lead to a loss of engagements, and a fall in public esteem. Although a flamboyant personality makes for good press, it is the steady and dependable performer who will succeed in the long run. In fact today's top artists are, for the most part, level-headed confident and hard-working professionals, who thrive in the intensely competitive milieu of the performing arts.

The performer's personality in response to the mood and receptiveness of each audience is also important. All members of the audience have now been exposed to radio, television and electronically enhanced recordings, and they expect much more of the performer than they did years ago. While vocal expectations have grown, the style of acting has turned towards more natural gestures and characterization. The exaggerated swoon or rage of previous generations looks ridiculous on video close-up. Especially in opera, the performer must not only entertain but convince their audience.

An actor or singer must be versatile not only because of public demand, but also because of the harsh reality of competition and insufficient work to support performers if the person is overly 'stereotyped'. Some of the best-known actors display this versatility to virtuosic level. The artist who cannot see the value of versatility not infrequently blames other people for his failure. The more versatile the performer is, the greater the chance of financial survival until the artist is sufficiently confident and established to choose his defining avenue for success. Part of a singer's aptitude lies in his ability to cover his areas of relative weakness. This is done by choosing appropriate roles, employing alternative technical devices, and recognizing that changes in the voice over the years demand a change in the repertoire. Persistent attempts to sing a younger artist's repertoire in the declining years will only hasten the inevitable decline of the voice. Examples of singers who have chosen their repertoire well include Joan Sutherland and Leontyne Price. Examples of the other group, those who 'sing off the capital, rather than the interest', unfortunately also abound and will remain nameless here.

5

General considerations before performance

Performance of a work represents the culmination of years of training and self discipline. Every artist lives for the opportunity to be heard, and wants to be heard at his or her best. Certain guidelines must be followed to achieve this aim.

The role which the artist undertakes should lie comfortably within his ability. The artist should know the part, as well as the parts of the other performers and the orchestral score. This gives a cushion of assurance during performance, and allows the performer to focus his energies on his own artistic effort.

It may be obvious, but the singer or actor should be in best possible health. Good diet, adequate rest and a rational exercise programme not only enhance a general sense of well-being but will also pay off in terms of stamina, particularly during a run of performances or on tour. It may be surprising to the lay reader, but most international artists live a simple, almost monastic life, which revolves around the theatre, departure lounge of airports and hotel rooms. Late night parties, excessive eating or drinking are, in the long run, not compatible with the demands for consistently high quality performance. Any free time is usually spent re-reading the script, or sitting in front of a keyboard and studying the score.

Vocal conservation is especially important. Singers and actors are usually extrovert and loquacious personalities. The touring artist finds herself in ever-changing surroundings, which necessitate a great deal of social contact at each new venue. It is therefore doubly difficult to avoid vocal overuse prior to the performance. Having made all essential arrangements with agents and management, the artist should cloister himself in his well-humidified room. If the available restaurants are noisy, it may be better to take a light evening meal in the room before retiring. A mild sleeping pill may be helpful, especially in combating jet lag or excessive performance anxiety. A short-acting hypnotic agent should be used, one which is not drying and free of after-effects.

Ideally, the artist should arrive one or two days before the performance, in order to acclimatize to his new surroundings. If the schedule begins with rehearsals, the performer should warm up carefully, and decide whether the rehearsal warrants singing at full voice or whether 'marking' will suffice. Dress rehearsals usually require that the performer sing, and it is, in fact, important for the artist to judge the acoustics of the theatre by doing so.

Conductors who are inconsiderate or do not have a good working knowledge of vocal production will sometimes require singers to rehearse for long, tiring hours. This is impossible for the very young performer and taxing even for the seasoned singer. Choral conductors who hold all-day workshops or long rehearsals are the most obvious offenders, for under such marathon conditions the singer can never perform at his best and not infrequently is unable to sing for several days afterwards.

The artist singing a major role should be reassured that a cover is rehearsed and available. An unfortunate practice of some theatre companies is to not begin rehearsing the cover until after opening night, usually for financial reasons. This puts additional stress on the artist. While at the theatre, the artist should also inspect the dressing room, and make a mental note regarding specific needs, such as a humidifier. Backstage areas are notorious harbingers of dust, debris and fungi, and the artist should stay in his dressing room as much as possible prior to appearing on stage.

The evening of the performance should be as free of extraneous stress as possible. The artist should be at the theatre well ahead of the required time. This not only avoids the anxiety of a last-minute dash across town, but leaves ample time to warm up, steam or otherwise hydrate the throat. It is the custom in musical theatre to build up to a crescendo of activity during final rehearsals and previews, which culminates in the official opening night. Management is often complicit in this flurry of activity, for reasons of publicity and lack of preparation. These artists must work even harder to maintain a sense of calm and equanimity at the opening. If the performer can remain in control of his environment and his own temperament, then on opening night he will be ready to conquer his audience.

To perform or not to perform?

Ideally, every performance should be undertaken when the artist is in peak condition. This unfortunately is more the exception than the rule and, in reality, many good performances are given by artists who are not at their best. An experienced performer is often able to compensate for minor problems, particularly if he has faced similar difficulties before. It is in fact the distinguishing mark of a professional to give a creditable performance even when he or she is 'under the weather'. It is therefore a large step from not feeling your best to cancelling a performance.

In weighing a cancellation, the physician's overriding concerns must always be for the health of the patient's voice, present and future, and for the continued good reputation of the performer. Enormous pressures can be put on by producers and directors, to get the artist to perform, for large amounts of money are frequently involved and a show may be built around a specific actor or singer. Even when this is not so, the performer always feels that he has a duty to his public and consequently a search is made by both the performer and management for a 'quick fix'. However, the laryngologist must forbid a performance that is liable to injure the larynx, for if the artist's condition degenerates, the performance with be ruined and the performer's reputation and self-confidence will be severely damaged.

On the other hand, reliability and a good health record are part of a performer's reputation. Frequent cancellations quickly result in fewer engagements and the physician should always make all reasonable efforts to 'keep the performer on stage'. Should a decision, however, be made to cancel the performance, then as much notice as possible should be given to find a substitute or reschedule the event.

In assessing whether the performance should go ahead, it is important for the laryngologist to know whether or not it is an opening night or part of a long run before giving an opinion. It is easier to cancel a single performance in the middle of a run, than an opening, or press night. Typically, also, the performer does not want to disappoint his public, and is also conscious of the expenses incurred by management. A great deal depends on the training and capability of a performer. Some voices can be devastated by a simple cold, while others, particularly in musical theatre, can sometimes sound better, especially during the early stages. The experienced performer knows how to modify style, diction and vocal technique and how to fine tune the script or score so that the performance will be acceptable. Popular music is more forgiving in this regard, since the singer can adjust amplification, make cuts and transpose his part to accommodate his temporary vocal limitations.

None the less, there are valid absolute and relative indications for cancellation. Acute laryngitis, with red and swollen vocal folds, will not permit a viable performance. This bacterial infection is often associated with a chest or sinus infection, and the patient's immune system is taxed in dealing with these problems. Singing or acting in this condition may lead to lingering problems. Vocal fold haemorrhage is another absolute contraindication to performance. In this condition, covered at length elsewhere, the artist experiences a sudden loss of voice which may be either painless or associated with localized one-sided throat discomfort. Complete voice rest is essential in this case, and continued singing may aggravate the haemorrhage, and cause laryngeal polyps to develop. Stage fright is not uncommon but, on rare occasions, can be excessive and virtually paralysing. If this cannot be overcome by reassurance or medications, the artist may be unable to go on stage.

Relative indications for cancelling are more controversial. If an artist has a full schedule of different commitments in the upcoming months, he may be inclined to cancel less important engagements to remain in top voice for that important premiere or recording. For example, a single recital in a less important venue may be sacrificed in favour of a career-advancing performance with an celebrated conductor.

While such situations may justify the occasional cancellation, it is important for an artist to not acquire a reputation for unreliability. This issue is further discussed in Chapter 7.

Illness before performance

Illness prior to a big performance is usually infectious in nature or an overuse injury. The performer may not have known his material well enough and has simply over-rehearsed. More commonly, however, there is a great deal of chopping and changing of material in the show as old material is taken out and new material introduced, learned, rehearsed, etc., to the point of exhaustion. An illness that is secondary to infection is more likely to have affected other members of the general community or cast, so that the physician will have some idea on how severe the condition is likely to be.

The larynx of a seasoned performer will indicate some variations from normal as would the hands of a professional gardener who has marked roughening of his palms. Even when the voice is at its best, some sopranos and tenors not infrequently have some mild soft nodule formation in the midpoints of the vibrating folds. Most of these are wide based and appear soft. A baritone/bass typically has large, reddened vocal folds, that suggest chronic laryngitis to the inexperienced examiner. These findings by themselves do not indicate illness or injury, and certainly should not be grounds for cancellation. All aspects, including vocal overuse, concurrent illness or psychological factors must be weighed. Ultimately, the physician must be the patient's advocate, and his advice, whether to perform or not, must be based not on financial or political pressure but on his wish to help the performer.

6

Laryngeal disorders: diagnosis, treatment and prevention

Introduction

The larynx is only one portion of the vocal mechanism, and the importance of the entire vocal tract, from the diaphragm through to the pharynx and mouth, has been alluded to, in Chapter 1 on structure and function. Clearly, medical disorders of any portion of the vocal tract will have an impact on the singing voice. For instance, chronic obstructive pulmonary disease, such as emphysema, will limit respiratory function, impede the free flow of air during inspiration and expiration, and decrease the ability to sing in a a loud, controlled and sustained fashion. Similarly, paralysis of the phrenic nerve, which innervates the diaphragm, will significantly impair the performer's ability to power the voice.

Even when looking only at the larynx, we need to be aware that any disorder which effects cartilage, muscle and nervous tissue may limit normal phonation. By way of example, Parkinsonism, a degenerative brain disorder which effects nerves and muscles, will often cause a deterioration of the voice. In fact, a complete review of all the diseases which may impact on vocal performance would probably require a textbook of medicine.

In order to keep this chapter relevant, we will focus only on disorders of the speaking and singing larynx which can develop in an otherwise healthy individual. In fact, the majority of laryngeal problems are benign lesions which affect the mucous membrane of the vocal folds. These disorders often develop as a consequence of vocal misuse or accidents and, once formed, will in turn dictate altered modes of vocal technique which may themselves become harmful. Structure and function are inextricably interrelated in the vocal performer's larynx.

The phonating larynx

In an earlier chapter, we have already discussed the phonatory mechanism. Certain aspects need to be amplified in order that the reader may understand how injuries develop.

Before the larynx makes a sound, air pressure must be built up in the upper trachea. This is achieved by pushing the vocal folds together (adducting), and exhaling. The folds are pressed against each other, and subglottic air pressure rises. At a certain point in time, the force of the air pressure is greater than the muscular forces pressing the vocal folds together. The folds are blown apart, and a puff or air escapes. This decreases the subglottic air pressure, and the muscular forces of the larynx temporarily gain the upper hand. The vocal folds adduct again. Pressure builds up once more, and the cycle repeats itself. A rapid series of tiny puffs of air is generated, and the frequency of this train of air puffs determines the pitch of the sound. Thus, if the frequency is 512 puffs per second, a middle C will sound. The turbulent nature of air flow results in a raw sound which is not a pure sine wave. It is modified and amplified in the supraglottic vocal tract, as has been discussed earlier.

Each vocal fold is made up of two segments: the anterior two-thirds of the fold (membranous portion) constitutes the vibrating portion, and is the segment that, functionally, is the phonating organ. The posterior one-third of each fold (cartilaginous portion) (See Plate 5) actually contains the vocal process of the arytenoid cartilage. These segments also approximate, but do not vibrate. They are responsible for adducting and abducting the membranous folds, somewhat like the sticks worked by a puppeteer.

Some textbooks discuss the vibrating vocal folds using the analogy of two elastic bands held taut and approximated. This comparison, however, is simplistic and in many ways incorrect. The vocal folds are layered in structure, and the superficial layer (mucosa) is rather loosely coupled to the underlying stiffer vocal ligament and muscle. Stroboscopic examination of the vocal folds during phonation reveals a smooth and rather elegant wave-like rolling motion of the mucous membrane. This mucosal wave depends on the ability of the mucous membrane to shift freely over the vocalis muscle and vocal ligament. The muscle and its covering ligament vibrate slightly, if at all. They are held firmly by the muscles of the arytenoid, the cricothyroid muscle, and the vocalis (thyroarytenoid) muscle itself. The attachment of the mucous membrane over the free margin of the vocal fold is loose. A thin and viscous layer (Reinke's space) separates the overlying mucosa from the vocal ligament. This layer acts like ball bearings, and allows the mucous membrane to roll back and forth with the flow of air through the glottic opening. The mucous membrane covering the vocal fold is in fact anchored only at the anterior commissure and the vocal process of the arytenoid posteriorly. An intact Reinke's space is therefore important to afford the mucosa adequate mobility. If Reinke's space is obliterated, either by disease or following surgery, the voice suffers.

In addition to a supple and unimpeded mucosal wave, the mucous membrane needs two other properties for good vocal function. The layer must be pliable, to allow easy stretching and complete recovery. While in chest voice the main mechanism involves the vocalis and arytenoid muscles, in head voice the position and tension of the vocal folds is controlled by the cricothyroid muscles. These elongate, thin, and approximate the vocal folds. Mucosa which is thickened, or scarred is unable to accommodate this action. Problems related to such injuries include difficulty in head voice, and particularly the inability to sustain a clean soft sound in the upper range of head register.

Finally, adequate lubrication of the vocal fold mucosa is essential for fine approximation and safe phonation over time. The cells of the mucous membrane of the vocal folds are unique. In structure, they are halfway between the mucous-producing tissues of the pharynx, and the squamous cells which make up skin. While this endows them with strength and resistance to injury, they also lack the ability of normal mucosa to generate lubrication.

Not only are the vocal folds unable to lubricate themselves, they are constantly in danger of drying, due to the rapid flow of air around them. The vocal folds are lubricated by glands located in the ventricle. A constant flow of watery mucus is necessary for normal phonation. As the folds are stretched and approximated, a microscopic film of mucus coats them. Inadequate or thick mucus will not only impair singing, but will also leave the vocal folds unprotected, and more vulnerable to injury.

Posturing abnormalities of the larynx

In the course of swallowing, the larynx rides up and down in the neck. This allows the larynx to fulfill its main function, which is to protect the windpipe and lungs from food. By rising, the larynx closes, and the back of the throat (hypopharynx) opens, so that food and liquids can stream around the larynx into the oesophagus. When the swallow is complete, respiration resumes, and the larynx descends again.

The upward movement of the larynx is reflexive, and certainly appears to be more important to individual survival than its downward motion. This reflex may be carried over into untrained singing. Singing with a high laryngeal position not only produces a thinner sound, but often is one feature of excessive laryngeal tension.

Similarly, the muscles closing (adducting) the vocal folds are more powerful than those opening (abducting), and excessive contraction of the adductors during phonation can also generate harmful muscular tension.

As in most of the body, the muscles of the larynx are arranged in two competing groups, agonists and antagonists. One group will elevate the larynx, another group depress it. One group will approximate (adduct) the vocal folds, another group separates (abducts) them. Part of the training of a singer is to learn to use these muscles selectively, contracting one group while relaxing the other. If both agonist and antagonist muscles are activated, an isometric contraction occurs with a great deal of tension but little movement.

In the larynx, the agonists and antagonists are not perfectly matched. If all of the muscles of the larynx are simultaneously contracted, the elevators will overpower the depressors, and the adductors will dominate the abductors. It is possible therefore to sing with excessive muscle tone in all of these muscles, but the result is a dominance of adductors and levators, producing a pushed and strained voice, and fatigue and discomfort in the neck. The larynx is high, and the three sphincters of the larynx are all contracted: the vocal folds are squeezed together, the false folds, epiglottis and aryepiglottic folds are all contracted. This results in the need for greater subglottic air pressure, and also changes the resonance of the supraglottic compartments. Over time, the singer develops excessive tension with pain, increasing fatigue, and possible injury to the vocal folds. Although the above description fits the extreme case, lesser degrees of muscle tension dysphonia (MTD) are often seen in conjunction with nodules, or as compensation for some earlier injury which has since resolved.

Acute and chronic laryngitis

The term 'laryngitis' refers to an inflammation of the larynx, nothing more or less. It does not distinguish between infection, allergy, changes due to vocal abuse, gastro-oesophageal reflux or postnasal drip. As a result, the term has become a catch-all diagnosis which reassures the patient but does not help in terms of prognosis or treatment.

Acute laryngitis is usually an infectious condition, although it may also be seen as part of an allergic response, or due to the inhalation of irritants. When infection-related, laryngitis usually develops following an upper respiratory infection typically starting as nasal congestion, pharyngitis and then loss of voice. Most of these cases are viral, although commonly a secondary bacterial infection develops once the tissues have been weakened. Uncommonly, the pharyngitis and laryngitis are bacterial, and then the loss of voice is accompanied by pain on swallowing or phonating. In cases of true bacterial infection, antibiotics and analgesic medications should be considered.

Although an acute bacterial infection of the larynx will result in red and swollen larynx, most cases of 'laryngitis' show surprisingly little change on visual examination of the vocal folds. Although the patient is aphonic, the vocal folds are close to normal, perhaps with only a slight erythema.

The true cause of aphonia in such viral laryngitis is a reactive elevation of the larynx due to inflammation and spasm of the pharyngeal muscles. The larynx is typically high, and the thyrohyoid space is contracted. By gently massaging this space and temporarily lowering the larynx, the patient's voice can be momentarily restored, although this will again disappear as the muscle contraction resumes.

There is no specific treatment for aphonia secondary to a 'viral laryngitis'. Some physicians have advocated hot beverages, massage to the neck or other methods of physical therapy aimed at relaxing the muscles of the pharynx and neck. In most cases, this is a self-limiting condition and the voice should return within 3–5 days. If aphonia persists for weeks, another cause, such as maladaptive posturing, should be sought.

Vocal rest

Any inflamed part such as a swollen ankle or elbow will benefit from rest. Total or absolute voice rest is usually justified for a short time in acute laryngitis, in vocal cord haemorrhage, in mucosal tears and after laryngeal surgery. However, absolute or total vocal rest – that is the use of a writing pad to communicate – is not usually justified for longer than four to five days. in fact, complete 'rest' of the vocal folds is not possible. Although the performer may be silent, the vocal folds come together during the swallowing mechanism, whether it be food or saliva, and they move with inspiration.

It is imperative that throat clearing and gargling should be avoided, especially during the stages of any inflammatory change. To request a performer to rest his or her voice for 4–6 weeks is foolish and totally impractical. Most performers would not be compliant and would compromise by developing a forced whisper which is almost as abusive as shouting. Partial or relative vocal rest means being economical with the voice, that is, using it only when absolutely necessary and when doing so making sure that the method of voice production is technically sound. Telephone calls should be monitored by an answering machine and only essential conversations should take place, and then only for short periods in a quiet, non-smoky environment. The performer should keep the throat moist during any conversation by sipping water and avoiding abusive throat clearing manoeuvres. A badge or sticker stating 'Laryngitis – I have to remain silent' is sometimes useful to convince rather verbose friends that they cannot take part in prolonged conversations.

As the singer is usually better trained for the singing voice than the speaking voice, a process of rehabilitation should begin by performing some gentle scales, avoiding the extreme upper and lower ends of their range. This will allow the performer to pace and control and even analyse the voice before speaking and is analogous to the loosening and stretching exercises that athletes carry out each day on waking. Singers should introduce the same principles of control and awareness that they use with their singing voice to their speaking voice.

A misconception exists that whistling is restful to the larynx. However, whistling is associated with the opening and closing of the vocal folds which is sometimes hard to distinguish from actual singing. The movement is generally somewhat jerky and is associated with poor breath and abdominal support and indeed may introduce technical errors as potentially damaging as poorly supported singing.

Modifying a rehearsal or 'marking' to conserve the voice is an accomplishment frequently neglected in routine voice teaching. Many performers when silently scanning their lines start vocalizing and this especially common when reading vocal scores. If a singer or actor finds his or her neck muscles tight and the throat tiring at the end of the 'silent reading' or listening, then sub-vocalization should be suspected. The slow and gradual rehabilitation of the 'injured larynx' is important and an increasing work load as with any injured muscle, is a gradual process. Even after a long holiday or a period of resting from production the vocal performer must make sure that before entering into the fray of the performing arts world he must undergo several days of gradual warming up well before the performance. No athletic coach would allow his prodigy to enter a race forty-eight hours after a period of prolonged rest without a carefully structured and gradual exercise programme beforehand.

Chronic laryngitis is a much less defined condition, one with multiple causes which often operate at the same time. The voice in chronic laryngitis is usually rough, pushed and pitched lower than usual.

This is the voice of news vendors, barrow boys, publicans, parade ground sergeant majors and many music hall artists. These people uses their voices excessively, too loudly and with a forceful or harsh mode of production. Not infrequently they smoke and drink excessively. This type of voice occurs most commonly in middle age, usually in males and has been characterized as the 'gin and midnight' voice.

Laryngeal examination in chronic laryngitis shows a spectrum of characteristic changes. The surface of the vocal fold is normally smooth, white and glistening by reflected light, showing very occasional pinkness from slightly dilated blood vessels.

In professional voice users there is some further increase in the pinkness which is accepted as being within the normal limits or at least physiological. Some vessels are not uncommonly seen in established singers, and are probably related to voice use. In some cases of chronic laryngitis, dilatation of vessels makes the vocal folds appear dusky red, their surface is slightly roughened and dull and their edges a little irregular. Punt has compared the difference in appearance to that of fine white or faintly rose pink slipper satin and rather rubbed red velvet. The pharynx and other parts of the larynx also show similar changes in the mucous membrane and there is usually an excess of rather sticky mucus. All degrees of the condition are encountered from slight congestion and roughening of the vocal fold surface to the well-marked stage indicated above.

Some degree of hoarseness and lowering of pitch of the speaking voice is to be expected as a result of the vocal fold thickening and roughening. Some actors are clever enough or fortunate enough to turn this to their own benefit, for although the voice loses its purity and clarity, it gains a characteristic, rich, huskiness which can be attractive. The effect in the baritone may be similar so long as the changes are not very marked, when an unpleasant, harsh or throaty tone results. In tenors however, the consequence is more serious, the purity of high notes being spoiled. The more the tenor, or light baritone, has been noted for the lyric, rather than the dramatic, quality of his tone, the more serious is the effect. The performer with these problems should avoid the consumption of tobacco and alcohol, especially spirits, and minimize vocal abuse. As a compromise he should remain silent for at least many hours before a performance for this period of vocal rest is likely to get him by.

If an artist's voice can only manage to get through six evenings and two matinees at a push, he has no right to accept a sudden Sunday engagement, although artists are very generous with their time and support for charity events. Performers with vocal problems should, when they leave the theatre on Saturday night practice total vocal rest or if that is not feasible, relative vocal rest, until they arrive again on Monday evening. The performer will be the gainer in the long run, although he will not understand this at the time the advice is given.

It must be stressed that the condition of the vocal muscles, which are always overstrained in such cases, is usually more important than the state of the vocal fold covering membrane. The possessor of a very powerful voice with less than perfect timbre can often find employment; but a weak voice in repeated danger of failing is useless, and no manager is likely to engage such a liability. Chronic oversinging, whether done to compensate for the effects of chronic laryngitis or an attempt to sing big roles for which the voice is not suited will, over time, lead to muscular fatigue with a wide wobbly vibrato that has no centre, and a voice which ultimately becomes off pitch and unattractive.

Mucus stranding between the anterior and middle thirds of the vocal folds is often indicative of vocal abuse. The mucus forms a bridge between points of maximal impact and, often, points of future node formation. Laryngeal dryness (laryngitis sicca) is associated with dehydration, mouth breathing, a dry atmosphere, and antihistamine therapy. Coughing and resulting inflammation may be due to deficiency of lubrication. However, copious thin secretions are better for a singer or actor than scant, thick secretions or excessive dryness. The performer with laryngitis must be kept well hydrated to maintain the desired moist character of the surface lining of the vocal folds.

As will be surmised from the above paragraphs, chronic laryngitis is a combination of many factors, including misuse, dryness, smoking and drinking. The appearance of the vocal folds varies, reflecting these different insults. The treatment is to unravel the contributing factors and address them individually.

Vocal nodules

Vocal nodules (Plate 8) are discrete areas of thickening along the vibrating margins of the vocal folds. Since vibration occurs only in the anterior two-thirds of each vocal fold, the midpoint of these segments becomes the point of maximal vibration, and the point of greatest potential trauma as the vocal folds contact each other. It is therefore not surprising that nodules typically develop here, at the junction of the anterior one-third and posterior two-thirds of the entire vocal fold.

Nodules vary in size, shape and appearance. They may be small discrete, white and pinhead-like in appearance in some cases. In others they may be large, flatter and pink. They invariably involve both folds, and the two sides appear similar, although not always identical.

The singer with nodules is most typically a soprano or a tenor. Lower voices do not require a prolonged and tight approximation of the vocal folds. While nodules occasionally form in the larynges of mezzos and baritones, these singers are not as bothered by the resultant voice change, since they do not use their larynges in the same way as the higher voices.

Nodules impair the ability of the vocal folds to approximate fully, and also limit the folds' ability to thin out (a function carried out by the cricothyroid muscle). They therefore cause most severe symptoms at the top of the voice. Singers with nodules have difficulty singing softly in high head voice. Loss of notes from the top, a breathy sound of escaping air as the voice is initiated, are two tell-tale signs that the folds are unable to come together. Difficulty in high chest voice, beginning the passaggio into head voice, is another feature of vocal fold swellings.

Nodules are not in themselves painful, but in order to close the gap created by the swellings, the singer may use excessive tension in approximating the vocal folds. This excessive muscular tension can create discomfort in the neck, particularly after strenuous or prolonged singing. Examination of the larynx may reveal obvious nodules. When the swellings are small, they may not be so clear. An hourglass shape of the glottic opening, or mucus stringing across the points of maximal vocal fold vibration are indicative of a problem.

Nodules are the result of repeated trauma, the consequence of vocal abuse. A homely but appropriate analogy compares vocal nodules to calluses of the feet. If you wears shoes that do not fit, you develops calluses; if you use a voice that does not fit, you develops nodules. Nodules are chronic phenomena. They will not form after one or two episodes of voice abuse, but usually result from months or years of poor vocal habits.

When nodules first develop, they show only as areas of soft swelling. With voice rest the swelling may subside, only to reemerge as abusive voice usage is again initiated. Sataloff has called these early changes physiological, and has suggested that they may not need treatment, as many do not progress to nodules. In any case, the transition between soft areas of acute localized swelling and true nodules is not clear. It is important to not frighten singers with the 'N word' after only one visit, particularly if the examination takes place shortly after an effortful performance. On the other hand, false reassurance in cases of recurrent or chronic hoarseness is also inappropriate. The diagnosis is made through a descriptive history and vocal examination as much as through a visual inspection.

Even with established nodules, there is typically an acute and a chronic component. With voice rest, the acute part of the swelling resolves, but the chronic part persists. Voice rest or medical treatment may be helpful in distinguishing these components, particularly if surgery is planned. Nodules need to be treated only if they cause a problem. While the operatic singer may experience difficulties with even small swellings, a rock or pop singer can often function with sizable nodules, at least for a while. The sexy or raunchy voice quality of their interpretation may be actually enhanced by nodules, and then becomes a desirable characteristic. These singers can often transpose music down into a more comfortable range, or use a microphone. They can further compensate by using a firmer attack and adducting the vocal folds with increased pressure.

Over time, however, the increased strain results in throat pain and fatigue. As the nodules increase, more pressure is required to squeeze the folds together, and a vicious cycle ensues. Even with great effort it may not be possible to approximate the vibrating edges, and the segments on either side of the nodules vibrate independently, producing a double pitch (diplophonia). Partial damping of the folds at the point where the nodules are in contact may produce a high-pitched squeal, analogous to damping a violin string to produce a harmonic. This sound, called 'the birdie voice' by Keidar, is abnormal, and diagnostic of a problem. Over time, the upper voice continues to be eroded, until, in many cases, the singer completely loses the head or falsetto voice. Since some popular singers have never developed this voice in the first place, using the belt for higher notes, the significance of the loss may not be appreciated

Treatment of nodules requires, first and foremost, a modification of voice use. The origin of the nodules may in some cases be traced back to a short period of singing on swollen folds. A singer may have had a two-week engagement which could not be cancelled. Pushing the voice when the folds are swollen may have engendered soft but definite localized swellings. As the singer tries to compensate by pushing further, she unwittingly embarks upon the road to nodules. In this group, the professional singer with solid technique, voice therapy is particularly useful. The benefits are less definite for the partially trained performer who may never have developed a seamless passaggio, or a clean, dependable and well-supported top. In these cases, therapy needs to teach, rather than remedy.

It is generally agreed, that voice therapy forms the first step in the management for nodules. Although not all nodules disappear with modified voice usage, proper phonation must be learned so that they will not recur following medical or surgical treatment. In some cases, the voice is so damaged that the therapist has 'no voice to work with'. In this rare instance, initial surgery may restore some voice, which the therapist can then continue to improve. Short periods of vocal rest may be of temporary benefit in reducing the acute component of swelling, but does not address the underlying problem, abusive vocal habits. Unless the singer unlearns these, the swellings will remain. Prolonged periods of vocal rest, stretching into weeks or months, constitutes cruel and unusual punishment which has no role in the management of vocal nodules.

Medical treatment centres around increased hydration, and reduction of inflammation. If the folds are dry, repeated trauma during phonation will more rapidly increase injury. A well hydrated larynx will have vocal folds that move and approximate with less effort.

Cortisone, either by mouth or by intramuscular injection, can help to reduce the acute component of vocal fold swellings. While cortisone has no place in the definitive management of nodules, some physicians may administer a short course if an unavoidable engagement makes performance mandatory. In any case, however, the performer should avoid continuous or frequent use of cortisone, since this will merely impair the body's inflammatory response, while not addressing the repeated and damaging trauma which triggers the response.

Therapy generally aims at reducing laryngeal tension by lowering the larynx, opening the pharynx, and increasing abdominal support of the voice. Not infrequently the cause of problems in the singing voice can be traced to a bad technique in the speaking voice. Many performers are somewhat extrovert characters with a loud voice that 'fits the part'. Voice therapy addresses these issues and some behavioural modification is frequently necessary. Therapy is usually beneficial, but not always curative. Retraining the voice of a singer, particularly in the rock or musical theatre arena, who wants to produce a certain sound may not be acceptable to either the artist or her management. Even in operatic singing, there is a premium placed on the pushed and intense voice, and a change in technique may trigger a negative response. The great mezzo Fiorenza Cossotto was once asked why she relies on her trademark pushed chest voice. She answered: 'Because that's what my audience wants to hear'.

Once a singer has optimally modified her technique into a less harmful method, surgery may have to be considered. Not every singer will require surgery, but if there is continued impairment, surgery may bring dramatic benefits. Even if the nodules are considered to be a surgical problem, preoperative therapy gives the singer the tools to prevent their recurrence. Surgery without therapy is usually only of temporary benefit, as the nodules will recur. This is not so for cysts or polyps, as will be discussed below.

Surgical treatment involves a brief procedure under general anaesthetic. A microscope is used to visualize the nodules under magnification. They are carefully removed using microscopic instruments. Removal is done superficially, staying above Reinke's space, and the normal tissues of the vocal fold are preserved. In our opinion, it is always better to remove a little less, even if it necessitates a second look, than to take too much. If too much tissue is excised, it cannot be replaced, and the result will be permanent or long-term vocal impairment.

Cysts of the vocal folds

Cysts are ovoid structures which lie within the substance of a vocal fold (Plate 9). They are lined either by mucous membrane or by skin, and contain either mucus or keratin flakes. Cysts are generally

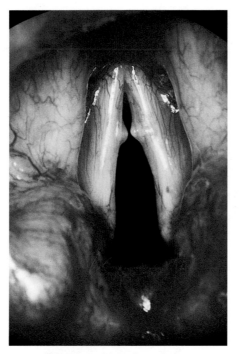

Plate 8 Vocal nodules

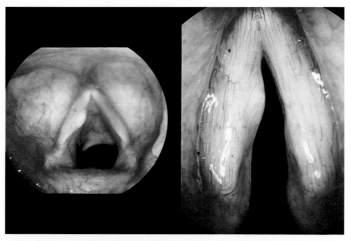

Plate 9 Cyst of focal folds

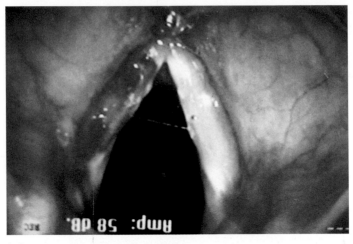

(a)

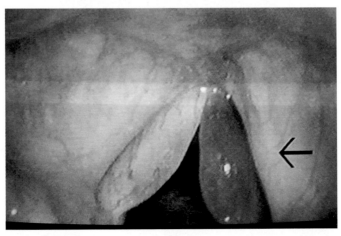

(b)

Plate 10(a) Acute vocal fold haemorrhage;
(b) Chronic vocal fold haemorrhage

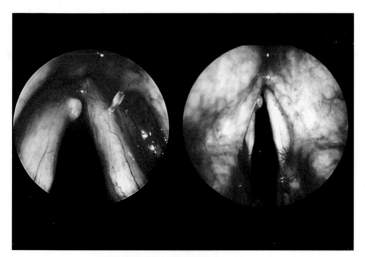

Plate 11 Vocal fold polyp

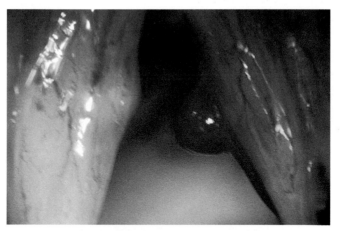

Plate 12 Haemorrhagic polyp

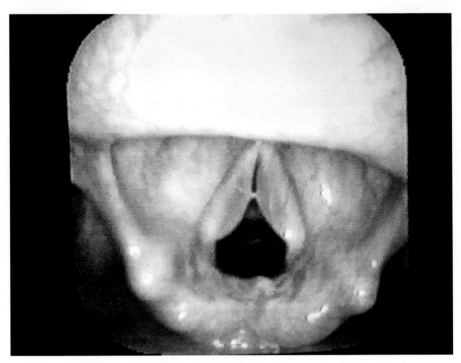

Plate 13 Diffuse polyps

less common than nodules, and they typically affect one vocal fold only. Cysts are usually the result of trauma: a bit of covering epithelium is driven under the surface of the vocal fold, where it continues to proliferate and produce mucus.

The symptoms produced by a cyst resemble those caused by nodules. The main differences are in their history, appearance, and clinical behaviour. While nodules result from chronic and repeated vocal abuse, a cyst can begin with just one episode of intense vocal trauma. In appearance, cysts are often confused with nodules. The main reason for this is the fact that a unilateral cyst invariably produces a reactive swelling of the opposite vocal fold at the point of contact. Superficially, therefore, the larynx presents with two swellings where the folds appose each other. It is only with magnification and stroboscopy that the differences can be appreciated. Unlike nodules, cysts do not respond to vocal therapy. They are encapsulated within the substance of the vocal fold, and have an existence which is now independent of vocal usage or conservation. Once the diagnosis of a cyst is made, therefore, surgical removal should be considered.

As is the case with nodules, cysts are only to be removed if they significantly impair the use of the voice. Housewives, office workers and factory employees may not be affected by a voice which is slightly husky and effortful. Singers, on the other hand, will be impaired, and will often have made the rounds of physicians, speech pathologists and others before the true nature of the condition is identified.

Vocal fold haemorrhage

The vocal folds, being living tissue, require a constant blood supply. Since the superficial membrane must float freely during phonation, the vessels to this layer do not come from the muscle, but run lengthwise from the anterior and posterior commissure. This arrangement gives the epithelium maximum mobility, and prevents tugging and tearing of the vessels as might occur if they coursed across the surface, or penetrated through Reinke's space. Despite this arrangement, the capillaries which supply the vocal fold surface are under considerable stress. The folds vibrate at high frequency and often at great intensity. The surface of the vocal fold is prone to drying, as discussed above. When a blood vessel ruptures, blood will flow out and spread under the surface of the epithelium, resulting in a vocal fold haemorrhage (Plate 10a and b).

When a vocal fold develops a haemorrhage, it becomes heavier and stiffer. The performer will therefore experience the sudden onset of hoarseness. The hoarseness may be slight or profound, but it is sudden and painless. Since in some cases the impairment is slight, there are certainly many more haemorrhages than are diagnosed by the physician: the singer may just note some hoarseness, which resolves after resting the voice for several days.

If the loss of voice is profound, however, the performer will often seek out a consultation. On examination, one vocal fold will be typically red and swollen. The condition is rarely bilateral. The area of haemorrhage may involve the entire vocal fold, or just one segment. If the haemorhage is not fresh, the colour of the vocal fold may be yellowish. Even after the blood has resorbed, there is often oedema of the vocal fold, which is slow to disappear. The oedema renders the fold stiff, and accounts for the complaint of persistent hoarseness despite no evidence of actual blood.

There are numerous proximate causes for vocal fold haemorrhage. Haemorrhage may develop following an acute rise in blood pressure in the head, usually with straining. In our practices, we have seen haemorrhage following coughing, vomiting, singing, childbirth and weight lifting. Among predisposing causes, however, haemorrhage is often linked to the menstrual cycle or to aspirin ingestion.

Most patients with this condition have had an associated upper respiratory tract infection or have been taking aspirin or other non-steroidal anti-inflammatory agents. Other blood thinners, niacin (vitamin B6) and cortisone should be avoided. Aspirin is found in a large number of over-the-counter preparations for colds, tickling coughs and influenza and not infrequently the performer has been taking them prior to seeing the laryngologist. Singers are often alternative medicine enthusiasts, and should be aware of 'natural' herbal concoctions. For example the Oriental 'tree ear' mushroom, a staple of Chinese vegetarian dishes, also decreases clotting.

In the case of women some form of oestrogen imbalance is not infrequently the cause of vocal cord haemorrhage. The mechanism responsible for voice changes during menstruation is likely to be an increase in the vibrating mass of the vocal fold as a result of an increase in its water content. Many women therefore notice vocal changes and difficulty singing during their menstrual periods. Female opera singers in the early part of the twentieth century were given 'courtesy days' and excused from performing during premenstrual and menstrual periods. There have been some suggestions that sex hormones play a role in modulating blood vessel wall activity, for spontaneous platelet aggregation is more often observed in young women on oral contraceptive pills than in controls. Although endogenous hormonal variations such as those that occur during menstruation may be associated with vocal cord haemorrhages, vocal cord fragility may be the result of the use of exogenous hormones.

The management of vocal fold haemorrhage is simple: complete vocal rest. Almost invariably, the blood will resorb spontaneously and full vocal function will recover if strict voice rest is instituted. The larynx is never truly 'at rest', since normal respiratory movements continue day and night. By avoiding forceful approximation of the folds, the singer decreases the possibility of recurrent haemorrhage, delayed reabsorption of blood, or the formation of a haemorrhagic polyp (see below).

Recurrent haemorrhage can usually be traced to a weakened blood vessel. This vessel is often obvious by its shape, size or location. At times, the vessel is hidden on the undersurface of the fold, and its presence must be inferred by its behaviour. While the presence of blood vessels on the vocal fold is not in itself cause for concern, dilated vessels or areas of excessive vascularity should be monitored. Not every vessel is suspect, and some asymmetry in distribution of vessels is not unusual. If, however, a vessel is dilated, tortuous or has formed a tiny blister (aneurysm), it often has weakened walls and is more fragile. Such vessels can be removed using a laser in combination with the technique described for nodules above. Obliterated vessels usually do not recur, although new ones may form if the larynx is predisposed to this.

Laryngeal polyps

Polyps are focal areas of redundant mucous membrane (Plate 11). They are filled with gelatinous tissue. Polyps are soft and, if of a certain size, may actually flip-flop in and out the glottic aperture with phonation. The voice is impaired but, unlike with nodules, the impairment is present at lower pitches. The voice may have a gravelly quality which is described as 'fry'. Patients with unilateral polyps have characteristic dysphonia. The normal vocal fold vibrates at one frequency, while the 'loaded' involved vocal cord dampens the vibration, resulting in hoarseness and breathiness, often accompanied by continuous throat clearing. Like nodules, the polyp also occupies the free margin of the vocal fold; at higher pitches, therefore the impairment becomes more like that found with nodules. Adding further to the confusion, early swellings at the 'site of predilection' (i.e. the point of maximal vibration) may be soft and polypoid, although in fact these will go on to form not polyps but nodules.

True polyps are usually unilateral, and in singers are most often caused by a haemorrhage that was not allowed to resolve completely. If the oedema which develops in a vocal fold following haemorrhage is not allowed to dissipate completely, an area of soft swelling will form at the vibrating margin, which over time becomes a polyp. These haemorrhagic polyps (Plate 12), like cysts, typically occur on one side only, however a contact reaction on the opposite fold is not uncommon. For this reason, polyps, particularly small and mature ones, are often misdiagnosed as nodules. This is unfortunate, since the implications of a polyp, in terms of treatment, are quite different from those of nodules. When a small polyp begins, any continued vocal abuse or misuse will irritate the area, contributing to its continued growth.

The appearance of a fresh polyp is often red or pink. It is soft and glistening in appearance. There may be a blood vessel feeding its base, although the vessel may be on the undersurface, and therefore not visible by outpatient examination. As the polyp matures, it can become firmer and smaller, and a contact reaction on the apposing vocal fold can develop, mimicking nodules. In more mature polyps, the feeding blood vessel may have scarred over and disappeared. Some polyps, particularly floppy ones with thin, tenuous stalks actually fall off, while others become fibrotic nubs of tissue.

Once again, voice therapy plays no role in the primary treatment of a polyp. Fresh and young polyps may involute spontaneously, and no treatment is needed, apart from modified voice rest. Some physicians will try a course of low-dose steroids to decrease the inflammation, and hasten resolution.

Once a polyp has been present for some time, it needs surgical removal. At the time of removal, the feeding vessel should be sought and obliterated with a laser. The contact reaction on the apposing vocal fold usually needs no treatment, and will resolve spontaneously once the irritant lesion is removed.

Diffuse polyps are an entirely different matter. These are usually caused by chronic heavy smoking. Hypothyroidism can also produce oedematous and thickened vocal folds and if this is suspected, thyroid function tests must be carried out. These very large, floppy (elephant ear), generalized, soft swellings of the vocal fold edges (Plate 13) are uncommon among classically trained singers, and seen more frequently among pop singers, radio and sports commentators, preachers and other professional voice users. Polypoid degeneration (also called smokers' polyposis and Reinke's oedema) is a diffuse swelling of both vocal folds. Excess gelatinous tissue is laid down in Reinke's space, perhaps as an attempt by the larynx to protect itself from the tar and debris which irritate the vocal folds day in and day out over many years. These polyps are bulky and floppy, and lower the pitch of the voice to a degree where a normal female speaker may be mistaken over the telephone for a male. The beginning, and *sine qua non*, of treating this condition is immediate and absolute cessation of smoking. If vocal abuse is found to be a significant contributing factor, this should also be forcefully addressed. However, not infrequently surgery is necessary for the swellings when they are gross. It is important to avoid stripping the vocal folds with surgery, Instead, microscopic incisions are made lateral to the vibrating edge and the oedematous material removed with gentle pressure and fine suction. Only one vocal fold is operated on at one sitting to prevent adhesions. A second vocal fold can be operated on, if necessary, 6–8 weeks later. It is essential to explain to the performer that his rather 'fruity' voice which is recognised as his signature will be altered and he may no longer be 'typecast' for certain roles. On the other hand, his voice will be more pitch-centred, and may gain in projection. It must be explained that his new sound after the surgery which results in a more normal vocal fold may no longer get him the parts that were almost automatically his. Therefore, the professional voice user must not only consider this himself, but discuss the matter with his agent.

Sulcus vocalis

This term refers to a furrow along the edge of the membranous vocal fold which becomes bowed to a greater or lesser extent. The problem is usually bilateral and roughly symmetrical, although sometimes the lesion is one-sided. The glottis does not close completely during phonation and forms a spindle-shaped chink. Histologically, the sulcus is located in the superficial layer of the lamina propria. The condition results in stiffness of the cover layer and is often associated with hoarseness, breathiness and decreased vocal efficiency. No long-term, ideal treatment is generally available.

Paralysis of the larynx

The two motor nerves of importance in phonation are the recurrent branch and the superior laryngeal branch of the vagus nerve. The recurrent nerve supplies the adductors and abductors of the vocal folds (the muscles which position the arytenoid cartilages), while the superior laryngeal branch innervates the cricothyroid muscle. Injury to either of these nerves will immediately affect the voice, and is potentially disastrous to the singer. The recurrent laryngeal nerve is most commonly injured during surgery of the thyroid gland, or as a result of trauma to the neck. Other causes, such as disease in the chest or the head, are also known. It can also occur spontaneously, most likely the result of a viral inflammation. The superior laryngeal nerve most commonly is affected by a viral or spontaneous paralysis. Loss of function of the recurrent laryngeal nerve produces a flaccid paralysis of the vocal fold. The vocal fold becomes floppy, and 'blows in the breeze' with attempted phonation. It loses both its tone and its movement, and is unable to approximate the contralateral vocal fold during phonation. The voice is hoarse, breathy and weak at all pitches. On examination, the paralysed vocal fold is usually obvious. There is no active movement seen on phonation, although some passive motion due to air flow may be present, and should not be misinterpreted as voluntary contraction. The arytenoid is usually tipped forward toward the laryngeal inlet.

If the superior laryngeal nerve is affected in isolation (i.e. the recurrent is working), the voice is acceptable at low and mid pitch. As the pitch is raised into head voice, however, the mechanics of the larynx become more and more dependent on the cricothyroid muscle, and this function is now missing on one side. The voice is therefore affected at higher pitches. On examination, the entire larynx rotates towards the functioning side, as the normal cricothyroid pulls the thyroid cartilage unopposed.

There is no treatment currently available which will aid in the recovery of nerve function in either of these conditions. In many cases, the nerve will recover spontaneously, and movement will return to the affected muscles. In other cases the reinnervation is faulty, and the paralysed fold will recover tone, but not movement. The normal side will usually compensate in cases of vocal fold paralysis. The unparalysed fold learns to approximate itself to the paralysed fold, actually crossing the midline to do so. As compensation continues, the quality of the voice improves, and may be, in practical terms, as good as normal, except when trying to compete with background noise. Since the clinical picture is one of hoarseness which gradually goes away, there are probably many more patients with compensated vocal fold paralysis than are ever diagnosed. With superior laryngeal nerve palsy, the recovery is even more difficult to monitor, but probably also occurs spontaneously in a large percentage of patients.

Paralysis in a singer is potentially disastrous, since even with recovery the voice may never be as good as before. We know of at least one singer with a congenitally paralysed vocal fold who has made a good career in popular music, but this is more the exception than the norm. Compensation following paralysis can be hastened with aggressive voice therapy. It is important to identify the cause of hoarseness in such patients, since voice rest is exactly the wrong approach in the treatment of paralysis. The voice must be pushed, so that the patient can develop the muscular effort needed to retrain the mobile vocal fold which must now 'do the work of two'. If vocal therapy fails, surgical modalities, such as injecting the paralysed fold with collagen, fat or other materials can be attempted. This bulks up the vocal fold, and gives the normal side a more solid edge to approximate against. The entire vocal fold can also be pushed medially by inserting a small shelf of cartilage or plastic through the thyroid cartilage. This procedure, medialization laryngoplasty, is accomplished be a small incision in the neck, and is usually done under local anaesthesia, so that the voice can be 'tuned' by optimally positioning the implant.

7

Anxiety, artistic temperament and the voice

Contrary to popular belief, singers and actors are seldom intrinsically neurotic – but they are very sensitive, working under circumstances which are physically difficult, mentally and emotionally demanding and tension-provoking. The artist has one skin less, to quote Benjamin Britten. He is hypersensitive to criticism and not infrequently superstitious.

None the less, vocalists and actors are generally hard working, ambitious, conscientious professionals who are particularly prone to self-imposed stress. There is enormous pressure for the performer to succeed night after night. If a comedian ceases to be funny and can no longer make an audience laugh, the money will stop – and very quickly too!

The lack of stability in a performer's life can also be disconcerting. The result is not only physical fatigue, but also a state of nervous exhaustion. There is little direct contact with close friends and family, for their 'support system' may be many thousands of miles away. Actors and singers expect an element of stress in performance, for this gives them a stimulating edge to perform well. However, when excessive stress and pressures dominate, then performance anxiety can cause major problems. Stress is sometimes aggravated by inadequate preparation and by the artist accepting work which he or she is not vocally prepared enough to sing. Even after the performance, a poor review, typically penned by an unqualified or vituperative critic, may continue to fuel the performer's self-lacerations. Stress is further exacerbated by agents, conductors, theatre management, teachers and parents. Such excessive demands can sometimes exceed a singer's vocal abilities. These circumstances may lead to vocal strain and ensuing dysphonia. As the stress factor increases, muscle tension also increases, and hyperfunction causes neck, shoulder and tongue tension, an increase in gastric acidity and also a higher incidence of reflux oesophagitis.

There is tremendous competition in the field of performing arts, and many actors pride themselves for being known as cooperative, and willing to go that extra mile. However, this malleability can pose stress problems and a sympathetic agent or director should be able to recognize this. Many fear that they will lose their jobs if they refuse to scream or to smoke on-stage or to use vocally abusive techniques.

All singers and actors experience some form of stage fright, particularly the inexperienced. The fear of being struck dumb, speechless or forgetting the notes or lines is a common dread. The fear of failure is then predominant and all rational thought tends to be clouded by this self-induced terror.

Stage fright can present as butterflies in the stomach, cold clammy palms, hot flushes, sweating, rapid heartbeat, a sensation of pain or tightness in the chest, muscle ache and tension, fatigue, jelly legs and dry mouth. Hyperventilation leading to dizziness, shortness of breath, tightness in the chest, nausea or a feeling of losing control can be experienced. A survey of over 100 actors working in the West End, carried out by the British Performing Arts Medicine Trust and Actors' Equity, revealed that 41% of actors become nervous before a performance to the degree that it has an adverse effect on their acting. Two out of three thought this became worse with age. Some 6% took medication and 11% regularly resorted to alcohol before a performance.

Even with such fears under control, the voice remains a sensitive barometer of stage anxiety. Singers are utterly dependent on their voice, and not infrequently stress manifests as vocal changes. The term psychogenic is often used to refer to vocal problems in which there is an alteration of the sound, but no observable change in the physical appearance of the vocal folds. There are, however, changes in how the singer positions and postures his larynx,which may be too high, or too compressed.

Hysterical hoarseness may present when a singer or actor is under extreme stress. The performer, very occasionally may become so frightened that acute hoarseness will even appear on the day before a performance.

Auditions are also a major source of stress. Actors feel that these are often arranged with little advance warning, and with no consideration for their working schedules. In the survey mentioned above, four out of five actors mentioned the general lack of courtesy shown to them as human beings. Young actors are often unprepared for the reality of auditioning and not getting a job, while older actors may take affront at being talked down to, and at the same time being discriminated against by virtue of their age.

If the stressed performer develops hoarseness, the vocal coach or teacher will sometimes find it hard to determine whether the problem is indeed entirely stress-induced, or has some structural basis. By providing the performer with a great deal of support and rationalizing the whole scenario, his confidence should return and the problem should resolve. It helps to breathe out slowly and think of calming images.

If self-sabotage takes place, the performer should work actively to increase self-esteem. Performers (and casting agents) remember their memorable performances for only a short time, but never forget the bad performances. At times of stress, the performers thoughts may morbidly turn to poor performances of the past.

If further reassurance is necessary, it is frequently helpful for the actor or singer to have a joint consultation with the laryngologist and voice therapist. If the larynx then appears normal he can be given full reassurance from the laryngologist and further advice from the therapist so that he can gain full confidence.

Physicians should always take time to see the singer or actor on stage in action whenever possible. The performer should not become a victim of medical jargon, used not infrequently to conceal an inflexibility and insensitivity and perhaps ignorance of the performer's physical and/or mental problems. In reassuring the patient, the physician must, none the less, listen to the artist's concerns, keeping in mind that the performer's understanding of his own voice is unsurpassed.

The vocal artist knows that his professional reputation, income and frequently, a large part of the fulfillment from life, depends on the health of his respiratory tract. He fears for the health of his larynx, worries that too many missed performances on account of throat trouble may injure his reputation for reliability and knows that permanent damage may one day result in the ruination of his voice and career. He then tries to analyse various sensations in the throat, often with erroneous ideas of structure and function for what he calls 'voice production'. He may well become obsessed with such notions which serve to increase his anxiety. He may then become tortured by fears, and the flames of insecurity may well be fanned by taking multiple opinions from fellow performers who not infrequently offer well meant but mythological advice.

In today's musical theatre, when the distinction between musical, operetta and opera is increasingly blurred, a legitimate operatic singer may be faced with pages of spoken dialogue, or an actor faced with vocally demanding, almost operatic music. The lack of experience, and technique, to deal with these new tasks can add to the stress of performance. Stress is usually a combination of interlinked physical and psychological components. For example, anxiety-related dryness of the vocal tract may result in slight voice change, and engenders additional anxiety. This can result in compensatory laryngeal posturing with increasing vocal fatigue and further voice change. The tension headache is well-recognized and muscle tension dysphonia associated with excessive neck and tongue activity may eventually lead to vocal nodules. Coffee, taken to overcome fatigue, and aspirin, taken to treat headache and muscle aches, both exacerbate gastric irritation.

In the frantic few weeks preceding major productions, actors and singers not infrequently develop generalized fatigue. This is due to a combination of physical and psychological stress. It is the price the performer pays for 'running on adrenaline'. If a body is physically tired, then its resistance to infection is decreased. Infections, in turn, make additional demands on the immune system, and a vicious cycle ensues.

Management of performance-related stress

To combat this sequence of events, it is essential that the performer has adequate rest and proper hydration and nutrition. Vitamins are beneficial, but should not be taken to excess, particularly fat-soluble vitamins (A, D and E), which may accumulate in the body to toxic levels. Water soluble vitamins (C and B complex) may be taken in larger doses. Appropriate physical exercise increases circulation to the muscles and vital organs, and generates a feeling of well-being.

Anxiety just before performing is a normal stimulant which the actor or singer should accept and welcome: it is this stimulus which produces a 'sharp' performance. However, when psychological pressures become severe enough to block or impair performance, counselling and stress management must be introduced, particularly if this is an ongoing problem. Anxious or depressed performers may have social, domestic or financial problems which are stressful, and which may not be recognized by management or their colleagues.

Difficulty in concentrating and chronic fatigue, when physical causes have been eliminated by the physician, can be a symptom of depression, and counselling and psychotropic medications can be helpful. It is important that the laryngologist recognizes the pressures that can exist in performance and not simply give the vocalist a pat on the back and say 'your vocal folds look great; it must be stress'. It is important to obtain a detailed career and social history as well as the obvious medical one in order to be able to advise the performer on future management of his problems.

It is during the discussion following examination that the laryngologist can help the performer sort out physical from psychological, avoiding unnecessary medications or cancellations. We find it helpful in this situation to show the performer visual images of his or her larynx, which helps to emphasize our observation that the singing mechanism is indeed normal and intact. A photograph is given to the patient for reassurance and future reference.

The decision of 'to sing or not to sing', as discussed in Chapter 5 (p. 29), is a joint one shared by the patient and the laryngologist. Both should do everything possible to get the artist through the performance, short of risking significant damage to the vocal mechanism. For an artist to miss a performance is a very serious matter, and the fortunes of a play or opera involving a great deal of money, the players' reputation and many people's incomes for months to come, may depend on getting a throat condition well in a few days rather than weeks. The laryngologist must obviously listen to the performer in this regard. Cancellations may be avoided if apparently insurmountable 'vocal' problems are accurately identified as psychological in nature, and effectively dealt with. A singer's anxiety regarding a specific performance is at times due not to that performance but the subsequent several weeks of a crowded schedule. Cancellation is a double-edged weapon. The artist who cancels frequently will acquire a reputation for unreliability which will, in the long term, surely affect his career. If, on the other hand, the performance is lacklustre, particularly at an opening or early in a run, bad reviews will return to plague both the artist and his physician. These are all issues that emerge during the course of an unhurried laryngological consultation.

With regard to vocal rest, this must be used sparingly and appropriately. Opinion has been expressed in the past, that there is no point in treatment of a vocal dysfunction caused by an upper respiratory tract infection or overuse of the voice, for the required therapy is to take 10 days rest from the theatre. Could any advice be more inappropriate to a committed performer, whose life and livelihood depends so much on the health of his throat and is understandably tense and worried about it? It is as helpful as advising a top baseball or rugby player or even the mother of a young family to take a week's holiday every time he or she 'catches a cold'. It is important that the vocal artist has a restful period before a performance and as much peace and quiet as possible between shows. Social vocalization, whether at gatherings, restaurants or on the telephone, should also be monitored. During a run, the performer should avoid noisy parties in smokey environments. Many second night performances are ruined by first night parties. One does not expect an athlete to spend 3 or 4 hours digging in the garden the night before a track event.

The performer may further raise his or her anxiety level by fortune telling, predicting failure and feeling that a bad performance is a foregone conclusion. By magnifying the apparent misery of the situation, the artist increases his anxiety. The situation worsens when the singer minimizes her talents, strengths and successes. Overgeneralization leaps from one or a few negative events to some iron clad rule such as 'I will never audition well'. Performers who habitually think in these ways will be plagued by doubts as they get ready to go on. Once a given doubt is laid to rest another one will crop up. The entire time prior to the performance is spent in a kind of cross examination with the performer acting both the parts of top prosecutor and terrified defendant.

Self-evaluation and management of performance anxiety

Occasionally, when anxiety has been largely alleviated, if dryness of the mouth persists, this can be helped by gently holding the tongue between the back (molar) teeth for a full minute, which can stimulate saliva production. Alternatively, sucking a lemon drop or the time honoured glycerine, lemon and honey pastille, or using an artificial saliva spray to wash away sticky mucus may be helpful. Various mucolytic agents can be prescribed by physicians to make the sticky secretions less tenacious and more watery.

Any senior business executive who is sent on a stress management course is immediately advised to cut any drinks containing caffeine. This includes strong tea, coffee and cola drinks. Caffeine may give a temporary boost, but long-term use mobilizes calcium from muscles and bones and leads to fatigue. Performers have been known to increase their anxiety to almost a fever pitch by consuming more than 20 cups of coffee a day. Once coffee-type drinks are removed performers become less irritable and a rapid pulse and heart beat tend to settle down. If a performer has a chronic coffee habit, reduction must be gradual to avoid a withdrawal headache.

The time to deal with performance anxiety is not 15 minutes before the curtain rises. Any technique for breathing, relaxation or self-affirmation should be well practised before this, so that it is almost second nature. Remember, the more anxious or stressed you are in the rest of your life the more likely you are to experience performance anxiety. In this regard it is crucial to embrace a general anxiety reduction programme to help you with all the stressors in your life. However, if the root causes of your performance anxiety are psychological in nature and are presently hidden, you will need to take the time to learn about them. No anxiety reducing technique is likely to work very well if you really do fear success or if your sense of embarrassment is activated every time you perform. The following long-term plan is designed with these considerations in mind.

The first step in putting into place a programme to deal with stress, is to ensure before accepting any contract that the work is well within your repertoire. It would be foolish to accept a commitment which is beyond your capabilities. A dancer who accepts a singing role in musical theatre with limited preparation and very little idea of vocal technique is going to be continually stressed and develop muscle tension dysphonia very soon.

Well-tried relaxation techniques such as yoga or meditation may be beneficial, as well as massage and the local application of heat to the back and neck muscles. If indeed the performer feels that his stress problems are being aggravated by a difficult director or conductor or problems with a fellow member of the cast, then, with the artist's permission, a diplomatic phone call by the physician to theatre management may be helpful as the honest broker in calming the troubled waters.

Psychological counselling and psychotherapy

Punt (1979) gave a tongue-in-cheek definition of the professional and the amateur by stating that whereas the former can do his job when he does not feel like it, the latter cannot, even when he does. Nevertheless, it takes an exceptional artist to endure emotional unrest, week in and week out, without his or her work suffering in the long run.

Anxiety is a natural emotion response to stressful events. In a performer it usually lasts just a few hours, but can last days or weeks. Very occasionally, it can be prolonged for years and interferes with normal everyday activities. The approaches most frequently used by physicians or clinical psychologists and community psychiatric nurses are either counselling, cognitive therapy or behavioural therapy.

Counselling which involves discussions with the patient and sometimes also the patient's family, aims to help the performer use his existing personal resources to deal with the symptoms of anxiety and resolve any life problems.

Cognitive therapy aims to teach the patient how to alter modes of thinking that aggravate and prolong anxiety. For example, anxious performers also often have palpitations and believe that these may herald a heart attack; by altering such beliefs, cognitive therapy can begin to reduce anxiety.

Behavioural therapy aims to teach patients how to replace unhelpful (maladaptive) ways of coping. If a patient can unlearn previous inappropriate patterns of thinking or behaving and acquire better ways of reacting to situations, anxiety may be relieved. Organizations such as the British Performing Arts Medicine Trust and Performing Arts Medicine organizations in the USA can offer experienced advisers and counsellors to help solve the anxiety problems of performing artists and use these methods as an alternative to drug therapy. Other techniques which are used are relaxation techniques, using cassette music and voice tapes, slow-deep breathing with shoulder relaxation. When practising deep breathing, care must be taken not to hyperventilate.

Medications, drugs and anxiety

Medications may have either a beneficial or deleterious effect on performing anxiety. Drugs which increase nervousness, elevate the heart rate and generally heighten anxiety include the decongestant pseudoephedrine and some asthma medications. Antihistamines, antidepressants, sedatives and motion sickness medications, while not anxiety engendering, can mimic the dry throat of anxiety and lead to vocal difficulties.

Medications such as the benzodiazepines have been widely used to reduce the symptoms of anxiety. If these drugs are used at all it should be with extreme caution and should never be administered for more than 4 weeks because of the risk of dependence.

Beta blockers have received a great deal of lay press for their apparent ability to reduce stage fright. Musicians, especially string players, have been helped by beta blockers such as propranolol hydrochloride in the past. Public speakers have also taken this drug. However, although they may well have a place in the treatment of tremor induced by excessive anxiety among musicians, most authorities feel that they should not be used indiscriminately in the treatment of performance anxiety among vocalists. Beta blockers are most effective if the symptoms experienced are primarily physiological, i.e. sweating, heart palpitations and tremors. They appear significantly less useful if the symptoms are psychological, such as fear, and anxiety. Some performers feel that taking this drug gives them a lack-lustre performance and they miss their 'sharp edge'. These drugs should only be used under medical supervision and the performer should try out the beta-blocker on more than one occasion, well before the concert, to determine accurately whether the benefits outweigh the disadvantages. It is by no means clear that these drugs can prevent tremor or palpitations without having detrimental effects on cognition, psychomotor activities and perception. A lowered sensitivity to anxiety and stress may also signify the lowering of feelings in other sensitive aspects such as emotion and musical expression. Beta blockers can have additional and potentially serious side-effects, including a low blood pressure, blood disorders, and in asthmatics, marked bronchospasm. In general, it makes sense to postpone using a beta-blocker until other forms of anxiety-reducing strategies have been tried.

Alcohol is a ubiquitous drug in the entertainment world, and drinking socially is generally accepted, even expected. Apart from the specific physiological effects of alcohol on the vocal tract, alcohol may become a crutch, helping to allay anxiety and overcome inhibition. Alcohol can appear to take the edge off anxiety but it will affect coordination, concentration and judgement. The danger of increasing the consumption of alcohol can result in a feeling of false courage and bravado and, as with beta blockers, the performer may well feel he has done splendidly, but his contribution on the night lacks lustre. Alcohol taken as a sedative to quieten the nerves or to settle the emotions, will sooner or later lead to excessive consumption and onward to disaster. Ingested alcohol is dispersed in the aqueous fluids of the body. Women are more likely to suffer from the effects of alcohol, because their bodies contain less water than men so that alcohol is more concentrated. Even when not performing, women should not drink more than 14 units per week nor men more than 21 units per week. Spirits are contraindicated and every glass of wine consumed should be followed by a glass of water. Some 50% of Japanese and other Asian people have a particularly low alcohol tolerance, since they lack adequate levels of the enzyme which metabolizes alcohol. Shortly after drinking, the affected individuals develop vasodilatation with facial flushing, hot sensations, rapid heartbeat and hypotension. These unpleasant experiences can act as a deterrent to drinking. It should also be mentioned that the complete oxidization of alcohol yields 7.1 calories per gram and some estimate that alcohol accounts for 10% of the total calorie intake in the USA. Alcoholics often obtain 50% of their calories in this way and soon develop serious nutritional deficiencies particularly for protein and many of the vitamin B complexes.

While some of the greatest singers were known drinkers (Jussi Bjoerling comes to mind), in general drinking and singing do not coexist comfortably. The damning label of 'unreliable' is given to a performer who imbibes before a performance and this label follows the performer in all concert halls.

The use of tobacco is extremely harmful to the lungs and the larynx. The performer who smokes to calm his or her nerves is responding to a nicotine addiction, which should be broken at the first opportune time.

Although the smoking of cannabis may give the performer a false sense of being 'at peace with the world', it irritates the pharynx and larynx even more than tobacco, and the damage may be permanent. Any 'friend' of a pop singer who recommends cannabis is recommending a shortened vocal life and performance failure. Cocaine, another fashionable recreational drug, has numerous cardiovascular and neurological effects which can cause serious health damage.

8

Popular music and the musical theatre

The vocal performer in the area of popular music brings different qualifications and makes different demands on the voice. Often, these artists lack rigorous classical training, and their vocal education consists of a few voice lessons, supplemented by vocal coaching. Much of their vocal technique comes from emulating other popular performers, including their idiosyncrasies and bad habits. The sounds they attempt to mimic are usually over-amplified and electronically enhanced, and often beyond the capabilities of the unaided larynx. Some performers are primarily dancers who also must sing to meet the demands of musicals. Some are singers who must also speak and lack the training to project the speaking voice efficiently.

The quality of singing voice sought in musicals and popular venues is radically different from that expected on the operatic stage. A pushed, belted voice, a husky and covered voice are not only appropriate, but essential for stage shows. Unfortunately, this type of voice production is potentially harmful, especially if the performer is not trained to sing effectively, and to recognize the danger signals of vocal abuse.

If operatic singers are the high jumpers of the vocal Olympics, Broadway or West End performers are its marathon runners. Eight shows a week, and runs of several months are common if the show is a hit. On their off-days, these stars are often found making recordings or personal appearances on radio and TV.

The Broadway/West End popular and rock musical milieu is a world of high wear and tear. Late night parties, smoke, alcohol and drugs can destroy not only the voice, but generally wear down even the hardiest constitution.

This chapter covers not only the voice-related problems in

popular music, but also some of the other aspects of working in this field.

It is not always easy to find a singing teacher for an aspiring pop singer. Many singing teachers teach as though every one who comes into their studio will, with some luck, have a career in opera and on the concert stage. While a background in classical techniques of voice production is important, in reality, approximately eight out of ten students that any singing teacher has in the studio will be in musical theatre or in one of the popular singing groups. Even those aspiring to a 'legitimate' career may spend their early years singing (and waitressing!) in night spots, where they belt Broadway hits over the clatter of dishes and the din of conversation, in an environment blue with cigarette smoke. The singing teaching profession should therefore develop some ideas on how to deal with the modern student – how to prepare them for this high pressure and abusive type of singing which attracts an audience measured in the hundreds of thousands, in contrast to the 2000 who sit in an opera house. The typical student must learn to sing show tunes, rock and other popular music with a minimum of danger to the vocal folds.

Many of today's top popular performers are well grounded in classical technique, and in tune with their vocal mechanism. They are consummate professionals who monitor their own performances critically, and have all the requisites to sustain a long and productive career. Others, however, are only partly trained. They may have been swept up by circumstances which have launched them, perhaps prematurely, into a highly visible and lucrative career. They lack the training and reserves to sustain the level of performance expected by their fans. The primary respiratory difference between trained and untrained singers is not a matter of total lung capacity, as people think. Rather, the trained singer learns to use a higher proportion of the air in his lungs, whereby decreasing his residual volume and increasing his respiratory efficiency. While sustaining a line on a single breath is most important in classical singing (such as Rossini or Handel), the ability to 'float' lines of a popular ballad is attractive and useful to the popular singer as well.

Posture is an often neglected but important difference between classical and popular vocal delivery. Classical singers, particular in choral or oratorio music, assume a stance which allows optimal breathing and phonation. In musicals, the song is often delivered with varying postures, meant to convey the excitement of the action. A musical number may be performed by a singer who is crouched, perched on scenery, or actually dancing across the stage. Even in a solo concert or night club, the usual posture of the popular singer may hinder optimal vocal delivery. Performers tend to put their heads back and place their microphone up to the sky. This alters the curvature of the cervical spine producing a tugging and pulling on the extrinsic neck muscles. The vocal quality is meant to show strain and suffering, and this adds to the emotional content and immediacy of the delivery. In addition to rock music, in a large part of British and American musical heritage, music is performed with this type of voice quality.

Belting

Belting is the name given to a pushed and strident type of singing. Described only half in jest as 'yelling set to music', it is in fact a loud chest voice which is forced up into head voice range. The quality of this voice is quite different from head voice, due in part to the fact that different laryngeal muscles are used. As discussed in Chapter 1 on Anatomy and Physiology, the vocal folds in chest voice are approximated using the arytenoid muscles and the vocalis (thyroarytenoid) muscle. In head register, these muscles are optimally contracted, and the cricothyroid muscle becomes dominant. As the voice rises in the head register, the cricothyroids contract, tensing and thinning the vocal folds.

In belting, the 'chest register' muscles continue to contract to a potentially harmful degree. In addition, belters, who often lack classical training, will also raise the larynx and increase muscle tension in the supraglottic area. On examination, the larynx is high, and the false vocal folds and aryepiglottic folds are contracted. The anteroposterior diameter of the larynx is narrowed and squeezed. This generalized contraction also involves the external muscles, between the larynx and the hyoid, as well as the strap muscles of the neck. This may, over time, lead to tenderness and pain in the neck.

The tension extends to breathing. Some belters lack 'support' for the voice, and use a glottic attack, both due to lack of training and for dramatic effect. Respiratory efficiency may also decrease, with the singer relying on thoracic rather than abdominal breathing, and virtually emptying the lungs due to inefficient breathing technique.

Singers who belt excessively have no laryngeal reserve, and are generally higher risk for inflammation, infection or injury. In the pop and rock singer who 'belts' a variety of changes can occur in the vibratory margins of the vocal folds. They consist initially of reddening and then the development of polyps and nodules and small haemorrhages due to vocal trauma. It is sometimes difficult to separate the laryngeal changes attributable to belting from the additive damage due to smoking tobacco or marijuana or drinking alcohol. Alcohol ingestion, along with late night meals can aggravate gastro-oesophageal reflux (GER), which can further irritate the vocal apparatus.

An unequivocal sign of faulty vocal technique, particularly in belters, is the presence of neck pain and tenderness. Palpation of the neck will confirm a high laryngeal position, with tenderness and spasm of the thyrohyoid muscle. The thyroid cartilage is normally a finger's breadth below the hyoid bone. In these singers, however, the thyrahoid space may not even be distinguishable on palpation.

Although a raised larynx may be a sign of poor laryngeal control, it is also at times necessary in order to produce the sound quality the singer seeks. It has been suggested that singing with a high larynx is not in itself harmful. In fact, many types of ethnic singing employ a thin, reedy voice produced by a high laryngeal position and no vibrato.

Raising the larynx results in shortening of the vocal tract with a subsequent raising of all formant frequencies, as well as a stiffening of vocal fold tissues that alters the vibratory pattern and increases fundamental frequency. There is a concomitant increased tendency for tight vocal fold closure.

As already mentioned, a raised larynx when used for a specific effect is not in itself pathological. The condition becomes harmful when the singer is unable to lower the larynx at will, and spasm develops in the extrinsic muscles.

Despite the ill effects of belting described above, singers need to continue to belt. It is expected that they produce this voice quality on stage, and substituting an operatic voice is unacceptable to both the audience and the management.

A great deal has been written about 'safe belting'. It is still debatable whether truly safe belting can be achieved on a sustained basis. Intermittent belting, using proper classical techniques of respiration and relaxation is in most cases not injurious. Classically trained singers usually have a rigorous warm-up routine, but this technique is not in general use among popular singers. A brief warm-up, consisting of a few scales to stretch and loosen the laryngeal muscles is helpful. Some singers prefer to do this in the shower, where additional advantages of warmth and humidity prevail.

Even if the performance demands a belted quality, the rehearsal may not. Popular singers may not be aware of 'marking', a technique well known to operatic performers. They should be cautioned to save the necessary but abusive type of voice production for performances only. One way to minimize vocal damage is to 'blend' the high chest voice into head voice. The blended belt has a different sound from the pure belt, but it is still often acceptable. To use this technique, the performer must, of course be able to sing in head voice, and many popular singers have never developed the head register. Those with vocal nodules are often so impaired that they have lost their head or falsetto, and are vocally restricted to chest voice only. If some regard the quality of belting as something less than culturally acceptable, it may be useful to remember that Rossini and other nineteenth-century classic composers had similar doubts about the early Verdi singers. Rossini felt sure that they were ruining their voices as they sang the 'band music' of the early Verdi operas. For him, as he pointed to the vibrato that came from their heavier singing, bel canto was already dead and their voices were already ruined. It could be postulated that in 100 years, singers may be taught belting techniques from the twentieth century in the same way that we now teach and prize the Verdi voices from the nineteenth century. Even in non-belting popular singers, technical problems may arise, due either to lack of training or the demands for a specific sound. Country and Western singers look for a 'twangy' hypernasal voice, produced in part by a high larynx and a pushed sound. Unlike in opera, where pure voice quality and controlled vibrato are demanded by a perfectionist audience, a pop singer does not need to produce a pure sound. Vocal harshness may even be desirable, as a way of conveying the singer's identity and lifestyle credentials.

Most importantly in popular music, the delivery must be meaningful and convincing, perhaps even more than in opera. On the operatic stage, the singer is aided by a dramatic plot, a supporting cast, sets, and a palette of orchestral colour. The popular singer must evoke the proper mood alone, aided only by a few instruments and visual effects. A husky, urgent, sexy voice may be needed to convey this mood, but this vocal production is taxing, its pitch centre often below the natural conversational frequency of the performer's voice.

Speaking is a routine part of musical theatre. Even popular singers in concert or in a night club are expected to talk between numbers. Noisy post-performance parties are part of the popular musical scene. These singers are no more trained for the speaking voice than operatic performers, but speech forms an essential part of their act. While in operatic recordings with dialogue (such as The Magic Flute, Der Freischütz, etc.) speaking parts are usually 'doubled' by professional actors, the popular singer is expected to deliver all of his own dialogue. His speaking voice, as his singing voice, is his 'signature'.

Management of the popular singer's voice

It is worth reiterating that much of the distinctive character, personality and identity of the performer relates to the uniqueness of the sound of his or her voice. That sound is often the product of a lifetime that includes vocal abuse, frequently abetted by smoking and drinking and rarely relieved by vocal training. Such voices repeatedly require medical help since they are unstable and give out under any stress or after any mild infection. The aim here is to get certain performers over the inability to perform without substantially changing the image of the voice. It is of no use to surgically create anatomically immaculate vocal folds if the patient's sound, which is his signature, has disappeared. A performer's reputation is built on a particular sound, which may be generated by a larynx with nodules, polyps or even false vocal fold activity. It is well known that Bing Crosby had vocal fold nodules, each one estimated to be worth several million dollars!

Although the pop artist works perhaps longer and harder than 'legitimate' singers, his repertoire is also in some ways more flexible and forgiving. A jazz or rock singer in vocal difficulty has the option to modify his programme, dropping more demanding numbers from the repertoire. The songs can also be transposed down so that they lie comfortably within his range, a technique almost impossible in opera. The singer is usually amplified, and suitable adjustments to the performer's microphone may overcome a temporary difficulty in projecting the voice. The flexible and forgiving nature of amplified singing is actually harmful in the long term, since popular singers may ignore and aggravate their vocal impairment until the voice is almost destroyed. By contrast, classical singers will discover their problem earlier, when the situation is still correctable. Performers are notoriously hesitant about using a cover or understudy, especially early on in the run. Management is often adamant, insisting that the name on the billboard appear without fail on the stage. If vocal difficulties occur, however, judicious use of a cover, especially for performances which are less important, is useful.

Amplification in popular music

A major feature of popular musical theatre is the microphone. Both performers and orchestra are invariably amplified, on Broadway as well as the West End. Many performers regard microphones as invaluable, and indeed some vocalists could not be heard without them. They are often a mixed blessing as entertainers are able to sing with a microphone even when their vocal equipment is so inadequate or out of condition that they should not do so. In addition, the modern trends for ever louder sound in many types of production sometimes result in the orchestra being overamplified, so that the performer, even with his own amplification, has to strain to be heard above it.

Singing on the half-voice into a microphone and obtaining volume by mechanical amplification does not result in the same timbre as singing with the full voice without such amplification. However, it is possible to get good tone and to some extent save the voice and this aid should be used to advantage. Furthermore, there is a class of singer who, by reason of a voice of small volume or some other limitation, is obliged to develop a microphone technique. Despite these constraints, such an artist may be a convincing interpreter and the results may be commercially successful.

The technique used with the microphone is different than that used in unamplified (operatic or concert hall) singing, and operatic singers who are on occasion amplified (such as at outdoor stadium concerts) may need to modify their technique as they move from the non-amplified to the amplified method, and back again.

Ideally, amplified performers should have small speakers (also called feedback speakers) to be able to monitor the sound. This allows them adjust their vocal output as well as their amplification, and helps to balance the sound level of the instruments. This is very helpful in both rock and musical theatre and, if not available, may lead to excessive vocal effort with resultant hyper-function, fatigue and damage. Monitor speakers are more often used by rock and pop groups than in musical theatre, and more readily available in North America than the UK. Personal ear-level monitors represent the latest and most effective way of tracking the sound mix of vocals and instruments. These are small devices similar in appearance to a hearing aid. They fit deeply into the ear canal and provide good fidelity. All sounds from the stage and some sounds from the audience are mixed by the sound engineer and fed by means of an FM signal into the ear monitor. The main advantage of this method is in keeping the overall sound level low and therefore safe.

When using the hand held or floor stand microphone, the distance between the mouth and the microphone is important. It is usually best to keep the microphone at chin rather than mouth level for this will prevent that occasional explosive sound that might occur if the performer stands too close and also avoids the audience from hearing when a breath is taken. There is no one distance from a microphone that is best for everyone or every situation, for voices vary a great deal as do amplifiers and microphones. Performers who work with microphones a lot have found that a distance of 15–30 cm (six to twelve inches) works well most of the time. If at that distance the voice is too soft or too loud, it is better to change the gain on the amplifier rather than trying to change the volume of the voice. Hand-held or body microphones are usually best for the performer.

Although well-trained singers and actors are careful to protect their voices, they may be somewhat lax regarding their hearing and subject their ears to unnecessary damage and thus threaten their careers. They depend on good hearing to match pitch, monitor vocal quality and provide direction for vocal adjustments during singing and provide feedback. Any problem with the conduction of sound to the inner ear (conductive hearing loss) such as wax, or fluid in the middle ear after a bad head cold, can result in the performer hearing his own voice more loudly, an effect he will tend to compensate for by singing or speaking more softly.

Hearing loss from the cumulative effect of environmental and social noise exposure has been called socio-acousis. It is essential that the performer takes steps to preserve the hearing by wearing adequate hearing protection, especially when carrying out noisy pursuits at home such as mowing the lawn at weekends and do-it-yourself tasks with power drills.

The addition of electronic amplifiers to music, usually of the pop variety, has led to much greater sound pressure levels than has been previously possible. Now the smallest group with its 200 watt amplifiers can make a more intense sound than 100 piece symphony orchestra. It is perhaps remarkable to think that, in a concert hall an audience of 2000 can hear a solo violinist without any form of amplification, but when in a room of less than a tenth of the size, a pop group requires amplification of an intensity that can be painful. The purpose of high intensity sound is to produce vegetative effects of a general kind, quite apart from imposing the sound on the listener. In order to have a musical 'trip' it seems necessary to have the sounds of a sufficiently high intensity to be above the 'safe levels'. Not infrequently, the mean noise level is in the region of 105–110 decibels, which is unacceptable from the audiological point of view. It may be that a level of approximately 95 decibels would satisfy both parties in being noisy enough to be enjoyable on the one hand and restrained enough to preserve normal hearing on the other.

The dominant feature of pop music is low tone, but this range, 250–500 Hertz, is amplified to its maximum. Fortunately, low frequency noise is less damaging to the inner ear than high tones.

The presentation of loud pop music is often interrupted by pauses which offer at least some possibility of recovery and exposure time is very different from that in industrial noise exposure. For listeners this will probably amount to two nights per weekend and for the pop musician an average of 18 hours per week exposure. Pop musicians with this sort of exposure time per week exceed the risk level and it is not surprising to find that between 13 and 30% develop a mild nerve deafness. It is also important to emphasize the possible harmful effects of listening to music with stereo headphones, for much higher sound levels are incident on the eardrum.

Unfortunately, the effects of noise and age on hearing are additive and a minor symptomatic hearing loss sustained early in the working career may become substantial when the effect of the normal ageing process is added later in life. The performer with an inner ear loss will tend to speak and sing more loudly because auditory feedback is reduced. The vast majority of perceptive or sensorineural loss produced by the ageing process, noise or hereditary factors cannot be cured by medical or surgical treatment. It is important therefore that a musician or performer is aware of his hearing deficit so appropriate adjustments can be made. A hearing test therefore should be an essential part of the performer's annual medical examination, for certain vocal problems could be attributed to inappropriate auditory monitoring of the sound produced.

The use of hearing conservation measures has also reached a degree of sophistication. Top rock groups routinely measure ambient sound levels, and the performers are often fitted with customized ear plugs which selectively filter the most damaging noise frequencies. The value of ear protection is also becoming recognized in the area of classical music. We are moving from the anecdotal flautist who is deafened by the trombone player over his left shoulder to a general concern of all classical instrumentalists regarding hearing loss. Hopefully, as differential sound filtering becomes more readily available, the use of these ear defenders, particularly in long and intense rehearsals, will see greater acceptance.

Projection of the spoken word is a special skill, quite distinct from singing. In theatres usually there is a dead spot in the back of the stalls under the circle. Often the first circle is quite difficult, whereas the upper circle or the Gods can be very good for sound, as the stage itself acts as a sounding board and throws the sound upwards. The acoustics of any theatre can be complex, and the quality of sound can vary, almost from seat to seat. There are always difficult places for sound in any theatre and actors become aware of this through experience. Sound projection depends on the kind of stage as well, whether it is open and thrust forward or recessed, and the degree to which the stage is raked. The structure and building materials used in construction of the theatre need also to be taken into account. The predominance of stone in a building, for example churches, amplifies all the resonance. It is the vowel sounds that are preferentially amplified, since vowel sounds are of longer wavelength, and tend to persist. Electronic amplification in this sort of venue therefore needs to increase the power of the consonant rather than to increase the overall volume.

A trained Shakespearean actor or opera singer can project his unamplified voice adequately to fill the entire theatre. The theatre itself is 'played' as an acoustic instrument. By focusing the voice down and using the floor as a sounding board actors and classical singers can throw the voice down and then bounce it back up. This is a traditional approach which may be more imagery than reality; none the less, those who have the opportunity to hear an opera singer on centre stage, while standing a few feet off in the wings will be surprised at how much smaller the voice sounds than out in the auditorium.

It is only by trying that the performer can find the best place to pitch or focus his voice. In such a setting it is useful to get someone to listen in at different parts of the theatre to find out what the results are. Although the acoustics of the empty theatre are quite different from those of a full house, this 'selective listening' helps to identify dead spots on stage, and may be a useful guide to adjusting the amplification.

Theatrical fog

In Broadway and West End musicals, there is an increasing trend toward special effects. Audiences fully expect to see the stage rise, a helicopter to land, and the chandelier to fall. Theatrical fog, once a 'special effect' is now part of almost every musical, and also some opera and ballet productions. Once used with impunity, some of these compounds are now recognized as potential health hazards.

There are different types of agents used to generate theatrical fogs and smoke, and these vary in potential toxicity. Symptoms of exposure to theatrical fogs and smokes include dry or irritated eyes, nose and throat, dizziness, headaches, upper respiratory tract congestion, coughing, blurred vision and nausea.

Occasionally an affected individual will fail to make the connection between these symptoms and the exposure, either because an employer has said that the fog and smoke were safe, or because the symptoms mimic those of other illnesses. Even more often the performers or technicians will not mention the special-effect hazards for fear of losing their jobs if they complain or appear unhealthy.

Exposure to these smoke and fog chemicals is not limited to professional actors and technicians. Theatrical productions from Broadway to school performances, discos and nightclubs together with amusement and theme parks also employ these products with increasing frequency. Dry ice is the safest material to use and is recommended, except in conditions where the carbon dioxide level would achieve intense concentration. Leaching or fuming inorganic chlorides such as ammonium, zinc or titanium chlorides have also been used. Of these, ammonium chloride is the least irritating and the other two should always be discouraged. Burning organic materials such as gums (frankincense), paper or resins, cause irritating smokes which are hazardous in high concentrations. Performers with respiratory problems and allergies and especially asthmatics, may be at increased risk from these smokes. Misting mixtures of water and organic chemicals such as glycerine, mineral oils, ethylene glycol and propylene glycol have also been employed and cause narcosis and mucous membrane irritation. The theatre doctor should be aware of the constituents in fog and smoke, particularly if his patients appear to be adversely affected by them. The physician should not rely solely on the product labels for this purpose as labels on most fog and smoke products will not list ingredients or will be overly reassuring. Some manufacturers label their products 'non-toxic' because they passed acute animal tests or because they assume that their customers are exposed only to small amounts on well ventilated stages and for short periods of time. However, most of the older theatres, especially in the United Kingdom are small, poorly aerated, with virtually no efficient ventilation or extractor fans. It is important that performers or technicians waiting in the wings should wear masks when they are at risk. Fogs and smokes thick enough to obscure vision may contain a significant concentration of chemicals especially if they are used in poorly aerated studios for long periods. Twelve-hour days are not uncommon during the filming of television commercials and videos. There is certainly room for further research in the field of theatrical fogs and smokes.

Travel and the vocal performer

For many singers and actors, travel is a way of life. Whether on extended tour with a theatrical company or flown in at the last minute from another continent, the vocal artist must contend with the varied hazards of travel, and specifically air travel. Apart from the usual discomforts and inconveniences of such trips, air travel holds specific problems for the vocal performer which must be recognized and dealt with.

Noise level on flights can be considerable. Engine noise is particularly significant during take-off and high-speed climb, but once cruising altitude is reached this noise decreases. However, noise level during mid-flight often remains high because of air turbulence and resulting vibration of the aircraft shell. This generates noise at the higher frequencies, within the range of normal speech. The aircraft's auxiliary systems, such as air conditioning, de-icing, defrosting, pressurization, also add to the background noise. In general sound pressure levels increase from the front to the rear of the aircraft, with window seats being noisier than the middle seats.

When attempting to converse against this background noise, the passenger's speech (the 'signal') must be louder than the background rumble ('noise'). For clear perception, signal must exceed noise by about 35 dB. Unwary passengers in this situation experience the Lombard effect: in order to be heard, they unwittingly raise their voices above this noise to maintain an adequate signal-to-noise ratio. The greater the noise level, the greater the intensity of speech, resulting in abnormal speech patterns. The larynx preparing to speak in a noisy environment will make muscular adjustments (pre-phonatory posturing) which may be appropriate for the ambient sound level, but result in excessive tension during phonation. In commercial multijet planes the overall sound pressure level at cruising altitudes is often greater than 80 dB. Some investigations have indicated that the level might be closer to 85–90 dB. Intelligible conversation in this situation must then be at and above the 110 dB level, tantamount to yelling or screaming. Quite apart from strain to the vocal apparatus, there is potential damage to the ears. The intensity of sound in such jets approaches the limits set by OSHA (Occupational Safety and Health Association) for safe maximum noise exposure: prolonged exposure to noise levels in excess of 85 dB in the work environment are believed over time to lead to hearing loss.

Speech becomes inefficient at this noise level and it is likely that 30% of passengers on flights exhibit abnormal speech patterns. In one study, abnormalities of phonation were observed in 80% of such noise-exposed subjects. Therefore, lecturers, politicians and other professional voice users who are likely to be asked to fulfill a commitment soon after arriving at their destination should rest their voice during commercial flights. If they have to speak, they ought to be very economical with the use of the voice. For safe air travel, singers and actors should rest the voice, even though the cabin seems quiet. Ear plugs decrease the background noise, and discourage a talkative neighbour. Feigning (or attempting) sleep is a useful ploy if one wishes to minimize unnecessary conversation.

Moisture level of air in the cabin is usually only between 5% and 10% relative humidity. The cabin air originates from external air that is drawn through the plane's jet engines, compressors, turbines, heat exchangers, water extractors and various other mechanical elements. The air is then conditioned and pressurized before introduction to the passenger cabin. Sadly however, in recent years many airlines only provide 50% fresh air because recycling stale air can save £50 000 ($75 000) per transatlantic trip.

Excessive voice use is doubly hazardous in this underhumidified environment. To reduce further dehydration, the singer should avoid alcohol, caffeine or sugared drinks. These substances are diuretics. Instead, copious amounts of water or weak tea should be sipped throughout the flight. Warm water with a dash of lemon or honey would seem suitable and the use of glycerin-based lozenges are helpful to keep the mouth moist by stimulating the flow of saliva. Menthol or minted lozenges should be avoided for they are particularly irritating.

Breathing through the nose is not only physiological but maximizes humidification of inhaled air. The function of the nose, apart from the sense of smell, is to warm and humidify the air. If the nose is functioning properly, by the time the air hits the posterior pharyngeal wall it is almost 100% humidified and at body temperature. The nasal mucosa further traps circulating particles of dust, pollen and other irritants, protecting the larynx and lower airways. Nasal 'air conditioning' during flight can be improved by the frequent use of a saline nasal spray. This is especially beneficial when flying with a cold, on antihistamines or other drying medications. If hot drinks are served, it is useful to make use of the steam from the drink and inhale it. The moisture laden vapour can help to provide some moisture to the dry upper respiratory tract.

The earliest signs of dehydration may set in after only a 3-hour flight. The nasal membranes become dry and the pharyngeal and laryngeal membranes also dry out, with the result that subsequent vocalization becomes difficult or even hazardous. Examination of the traveller's larynx may reveal loss of the normal glistening appearance, and the presence of thick, mucoid secretions on the posterior pharyngeal wall. The vocal folds themselves appear dry, with clumps of white mucus on the surface, sometimes forming a string-like bridge across the points of maximal vibration. On a long flight the singer may, at the risk of social ostracism, consider wearing a surgical mask and placing one or two moist paper tissues inside this so that moistened air enters the nose and throat when dozing or sleeping.

The professional voice user should avoid, whenever possible, travelling with a head cold. Eustachian tube dysfunction, either due to a cold, or to other factors, results in ear pain and hearing loss. It can be largely prevented by the use of a long-acting nasal preparation such as Otrivine, or Afrin. Pressure equalizing ear plugs, recently introduced, may be helpful. In flight, passenger cabins are often chilly, averaging between 20 and 22.2° Celsius (68–72° Fahrenheit). Cabin and cockpit crews prefer the cooler temperature, which is more comfortable for work. Sedentary passengers, however, find such temperatures uncomfortable. To avoid a chill, the passenger should dress in layers, so that items of clothing may be added or removed as the temperature dictates. Mindful of the general drop in body temperature with sleep, the singer should make sure there is an adequate supply of blankets, especially for intercontinental flights.

As well as being annoying, environmental tobacco smoke has been cited as a cause of in-flight headaches, eye, nose and throat irritation, and breathing problems. Although segregation of passengers who smoke seems to be reasonably effective in reducing complaints about environmental tobacco smoke during flights, a total ban of smoking on all aircrafts would be the obvious answer. Several major carriers have recently instituted such a ban, however smaller airlines, especially in Eastern Europe, are more lax in this regard. The singer should always inquire about the smoking policy on any flight before booking, and insist on being seated as far away from the smoking section as possible if a non-smoking flight is not an option.

While the quality of cabin air is a major hazard to the vocal tract, the general malaise associated with air travel is multi-factorial in nature. Jet lag is probably mostly due to the effect of time zone change on the circadian rhythm. This is less problematic on day flights, and on travelling east to west. The circadian clock can be more smoothly 're-set' by avoiding caffeine before the flight, and eating a high carbohydrate meal in the evening, followed by a high protein breakfast. The recent interest in melatonin is due in part to this chemical's apparent ability to ease jet lag.

Other causes of fatigue, such as the motion of the aircraft, jet lag and even difficulties associated with airport procedures cannot be ignored. All of these stress factors not only adversely affect the voice, but generally lower the immune resistance, leaving the singer more vulnerable to respiratory tract infections.

If possible, the internationally travelling artist should arrive early, in order to allow at least 24 hours of rest before any difficult performance or rehearsal. On arrival, he should go to his hotel and actively rehydrate before retiring. Rehydration involves drinking copious amounts of water and making sure his room is well humidified. This can be done by filling the tub with hot water, or running a hot shower with the bathroom door open. A light meal without alcohol, preferably taken in the room or alone, is followed by rest, before appearing 'officially' the following day. Most popular musical performers, particularly those on national tours, travel by bus rather than aircraft. Many of the problems inherent in air travel are also found here, particularly the danger of excessive voice use over a background of motor and tyre noise pollution. The air in an air-conditioned bus is dry, and if the traffic is congested, pollution from the exhaust and other vehicles is drawn into the cabin. Many pop artists smoke, and smoke of both the tobacco and marijuana variety is freely generated by both musicians and road crew. Some performers sing and rehearse on the bus, and are again in danger of excessive voice use due to the Lombard effect.

To summarize travel-related issues, the performer should be well rested and in optimal health. If a trip can be planned, it should involve a day flight, with resting on the flight, minimal conversation and adequate hydration. Upon arrival, the performer should rest, hydrate and reset the internal clock as much as possible before arriving at the theatre.

10

Medications and the professional voice

Introduction

Medications are a ubiquitous part of life, whether taken by prescription, over the counter or for social reasons. For our purposes, any material taken internally should be evaluated for side-effects potentially affecting the vocal tract and the voice.

Singing and professional speaking require a series of highly coordinated neuromuscular activities, involving the central and peripheral nervous system as well as the muscles of the abdomen, chest, neck and larynx. While some of these muscles are required for slow gradual contraction, others must move rapidly, repeatedly and without fatigue. The mucous membranes of the larynx and pharynx must be moist and supple for proper phonation. The circulation to these areas is vital for proper tissue metabolism, and blood vessels must be ample, capable and resilient. The above brief outline touches on the major areas which may be affected by medications, either as an intended result, or as an unintended side-effect of treatment.

For proper function of the vocal folds, there must be a constant flow of thin mucus which coats the larynx. While mucus is freely produced in the back of the throat, the vocal folds themselves lack mucous glands. They depend for lubrication on mucus secreted by the lining of the ventricles, pockets which separate the false and the true folds.

Normal voice production depends on the presence of an uninhibited movement, 'virtually a flow', of vocal fold mucosa (cover) over the vocal ligament (body). Hydration is therefore important, both for the formation of mucus to coat the vocal folds, and for the internal lubrication which facilitates free gliding of the cover over the body of the vocal fold. If the lubrication of the vocal fold is lacking, phonation will be affected. If secretions become more tenacious and sticky, vocal problems may develop. The laryngologist must therefore be aware of any side-effects of prescribed drugs.

In the absence of lubricating mucus, the folds are unable to approximate properly. This is particularly noticeable in the soft phonation of high notes. If the mucus is too viscid, it forms clumps which cause an irregular fry-like voice that, if dehydration is severe, almost sounds like vocal fold polyps. In addition to an adequate film of thin mucus, the mucous membrane (epithelium) of the vocal fords must oscillate freely over the underlying vocal ligament and muscle. This requires adequate systemic hydration.

Medications can interfere with this mechanism in two ways. They can inhibit mucus secretion and flow over the surface of the fold, and they can cause dehydration, resulting in improper oscillation of the vocal fold epithelium.

Antihistamines represent the largest group of drugs which decrease mucus formation. Several over-the-counter cold medications contain decongestants as well as antihistamines. These medications are ubiquitous, and freely taken, especially in the allergy season. The antihistamine may well be drying the secretion and the decongestant will usually thicken secretions on the laryngeal surface. Many cough suppressant mixtures often include agents that have a secondary drying effect on laryngeal secretions, especially those containing codeine. Other OTC (over-the-counter) preparations, such as dextromethorphan, have pharmacological effects similar to those of codeine and form the basis of many cough suppressant mixtures. Antihistamines are also taken specifically for inhalant allergies, or for an acute allergic reaction, such as hives. Other drugs which act in the same way are the anti-emetics, taken for motion sickness, vertigo and nausea, as well as some antidepressants. The singer who needs antihistamines should experiment to find the medication which gives the most benefit with the least drying. Some newer antihistamines such as cetirizine dihydrochlor (Zirtek) or loratadine (Clarityn) produce less drowsiness and often less dryness, but in allergic conditions they are less effective than drugs with more marked sedation. There is significant variation in how patients react to a particular antihistamine, and performers should therefore tell the physician if, based on past experience, they prefer one medication over another.

In general, the singer on antihistamines should increase his fluid intake, and beware of combination 'cold-and-flu' type medications which often include three or even more different drugs, all drying and sedating. It must be stressed that the recommended dose of any drug is only a guide and there is individual variability in response and sensitivity.

Drugs that dry upper respiratory tract secretions are numerous. Many current antihypertensive agents have a secondary dehydrating effect on the mucous membrane of the upper respiratory tract. Diuretics, usually taken to treat hypertension or congestive heart disease, act to drive sodium-bound water out of the body, also causing dryness. ACE inhibitors are better tolerated than methyldopa and non-selective beta-blockers, but their long-term effects are not yet known. They cause a dry tickling cough in 10–25% of those taking them. However, since these medications treat a chronic and potentially serious problem, their use should not be discontinued for relatively less important reasons. If, on the other hand, less drying drugs of equal efficacy can be substituted by the physician, there is an advantage to the singer.

Some drugs used for depression can also dry the throat, and if troublesome the prescribing physician may well have to search for an alternative suitable medication. Large doses of vitamin C taken in an effort to prevent common colds, may cause excessive urination, resulting in drying of the vocal tract.

More detailed information on drug side-effects should be obtained from the pharmacist.

The viscosity of upper respiratory tract secretions is also increased by environmental dryness. Insensible water loss, mainly through exhalation, is greater in the winter, with cold dry weather outside and overheated rooms indoors. The ideal moisturizing agent for the respiratory tract is water in the form of increased fluid intake and a raised environmental humidity. A useful guide is for the performer to drink two glasses of water with each meal and one between each meal. Juices, tea, coffee or sodas are not acceptable substitutes for water. These drinks contain either sugar or caffeine, both of which act as diuretics. The third commonly ingested diuretic is, of course, alcohol. Not only do these drinks not replace water, but they actually promote dehydration through diuresis. Even decaffeinated tea or coffee contains caffeine, although in smaller amounts.

While it is usually not necessary to avoid a moderate intake of these beverages, the only acceptable water substitute for a singer is caffeine-free herbal tea. Artificial saliva substitutes such as Salivart and Glandosane are generally available as a mouth sprays or as drops, and are helpful to combat dryness of the mouth, but do not replenish moisture in the larynx or trachea. Another group of substances which can cause drying of the upper respiratory tract are the topical decongestants used to treat nasal blockage. These medications act by shrinking the blood vessels to the mucous membranes, and thus diminish the secretory activity of the mucous glands.

A skilful vocal performance requires the fine coordination of the laryngeal muscles, and any drug that alters sensation or coordination will, in turn, adversely affect these functions. Van Lawrence has used the analogy of the voice being akin to a musical instrument, and draws a parallel to a piano player who would be greatly handicapped by wearing cotton gloves at a performance. The professional voice user would be similarly impeded if pharmacological agents inhibited the perception of sensation from laryngeal pressure receptors.

Sedatives and tranquillizers are all central nervous system depressants and dull the senses. Alcohol is probably the most commonly used drug in this category. These drugs deprive the artist of his or her sharpness of wit and the sparkle of a great performance. Nevertheless, there is a great demand for their use in view of the hectic schedule of many professionals. It may seem on occasion that their use is appropriate, i.e. to provide a good night's sleep after intercontinental flights. However, problems occur when it is time to perform and the performance for the artist may be sluggish rather than sharp and alert. The person then requires a stimulant and after the performance requests a further sedative so that he can relax once more. Thus, the vicious cycle continues. Careers and even lives have been destroyed by the misuse of these drugs and it is far wiser for the performer to plan a less hectic schedule and also to seek counselling and advice regarding anxiety in performance and sleep disturbance problems.

Corticosteroid preparations may affect protein bound water in the vocal folds and have a limited role when used specifically and sparingly to reduce swelling or oedema of the vocal folds. Because of their anti-inflammatory action, corticosteroids are also used as decongestants. In an acute situation where one time administration is all that is required, steroids are relatively safe, provided there are no medical contraindications. If the patient has a concurrent infection, it should be 'covered' by the appropriate antibiotic therapy. It is important strongly to emphasize that steroids should not be used as chronic vocal decongestants over long periods of time. They are for emergency treatment only and then are used in short, sharp doses. They cannot safely or effectively cover a prolonged 'run' of performances over several weeks.

Steroids should not be used prior to any important performance unless the performer has used them previously and knows how his or her voice will react to them. An unpredictable, even disastrous effect may result from the emergency use of steroids to reduce or prevent laryngeal swelling. The process of 'warming up' may be inhibited so that the voice remains thin and weak, forcing the performer to strive even harder to achieve the feel and sound to which he or she is accustomed. Some general practitioners give performers 50 or more tablets of prednisolone with instructions to take 5 mg or so when the need arises. This is bad medical practice, since it does not address the specific circumstances of each situation. For example, a singer may have become hoarse from a haemorrhage which goes undiagnosed. This will be unresponsive to steroids, and will give the performer a false sense of security while furthering the damage.

Corticosteroid inhalant sprays may be occasionally beneficial for hoarseness, however, their main role is for prophylaxis in adult asthma. These inhaled corticosteroids are usually well tolerated, but when used for long periods they may well result in Candida laryngitis, as discussed elsewhere. Thrush in the mouth and pharynx occurs in over 30% of adults who use these inhalers on a regular basis. The incidence of oral and pharyngeal thrush may be reduced with spacer devices and also by rinsing and gargling after the use of the spray. Dysphonia occurs in up to 50% of patients using steroid inhalers and it is related to the aerosol steroid itself rather than the propellant. Prolonged steroid use which is common in asthmatics is also believed by some to cause possible wasting of the vocalis muscle (steroid-related myopathy). Examination of such a patient will disclose vocal folds which are thinner and which fail to meet properly upon phonation. Treatment should be stopped if there is hoarseness due either to wasting or thrush and appropriate treatment of infection with institution of an alternative asthma medication should be considered. Dysphonia may at times be avoided if a lower dose of inhaled steroids is tried.

Mucolytic agents supplement humidification by assisting bronchial drainage and also reduce the amount of coughing necessary to clear the bronchi. Iodinated glycerol is effective, but should be used sparingly and is not trouble free, although the iodine content has been drastically reduced. Even so, it is important to check for iodine sensitivity, and monitor thyroid function. Preparations containing guiafenesin are now replacing the iodinated glycerol preparations. Throat sprays have occupied a traditional place in the laryngologist's domiciliary bag, when visiting performers backstage. Many of these time-honoured sprays however, contain harmful substances. Any preparation which is applied directly to the throat can have troublesome side-effects and classical preparations such as diphenhydramine hydrochloride (Benadryl) 9% in water, has a distinct local anaesthetic effect. The so-called Lady Melba spray also falls into this group, and is not recommended. The very occasional use of oxymetazoline (Afrin or Afrazine) may be helpful, but water is safest and should always prove helpful particularly in cases of excessive dryness of the larynx. Throat lozenges should be non-medicated and as bland as possible. Allen and Hanbury's glycerine, blackcurrant and honey pastilles or Pine Brothers honey and glycerine tablets are both innocuous and useful. Water or saline delivered via a vaporizer or steam generator, is frequently effective and sufficient. Normal (isotonic) saline, applied with a small perfume-type atomizer makes the ideal portable lubricant. As already discussed in the section on travel, a performer on entering his room in a high rise hotel should immediately run the shower with the hottest water and allow the steam to circulate into his room even before unpacking his suitcase. On return from the theatre at night the same process should be repeated. Many actors and singers carry small hand-held humidifiers in their travel kit.

A simple normal saline spray also can be helpful to clear thick debris from the back of the nose. Post-nasal drip may accumulate for a number of reasons, including allergy, infection or nasal obstruction. As this material drips down into the throat, pharyngitis, tonsillitis and laryngeal problems may result. The nasal cavities can be more systematically cleared using saline instilled by means of a nasal douche. The Birmingham type of nasal douche is useful. Equally effective is a Neti pot, often used before yoga and meditation, and available at alternative health stores. Physicians who treat patients for upper respiratory tract infections with tracheitis, pharyngitis and laryngitis will quite frequently, prescribe gargles using salt water and solutions of aspirin. Although aspirin and other salycilate-containing preparations may be useful, they also facilitate bleeding by interfering with clotting. None the less, aspirin may be the preferred medication for a range of conditions such as arthritis, the common cold, aches and pains and hangover cures. Singers and actors not infrequently perform in concert halls and theatres with low humidity and this causes marked dryness of the nose. Forcible blowing of the nose in a patient taking aspirin may induce a troublesome nosebleed. Vocal fold haemorrhage, a potentially catastrophic situation, is promoted by aspirin ingestion, and is covered in greater detail elsewhere. Thus, for any minor ailment where aspirin is usually indicated, alternative preparations such as paracetamol should be considered. Aspirin preparations should be discontinued for 7–10 days prior to any form of surgery.

Non-steroidal anti-inflammatory drugs (NSAIDs) can, when used with an inflamed throat, also increase the risk of haemorrhage into the vocal folds. Nose bleeds can also be associated with the use of this group of drugs. All of these medications increase gastric acidity and the tendency for gastro-oesphageal reflux disorders (GERD). These conditions are covered elsewhere in the text.

The use of gargles for inflammatory conditions in the larynx and pharynx is time honoured, but has little or no scientific validity. Scientific studies with a radio-opaque gargling medium have shown that the typical gargle goes back no further than the tonisillar pillars, and does not have any direct contact with the hypopharynx or larynx. Gargling with a warm liquid may have a slight generalized benefit in inducing hyperaemia (increased blood circulation) to the mucous membranes. On the other hand, gargling may be traumatic and irritating to the vocal mechanism, causing a firm and harsh arytenoid compression, especially in patients with laryngitis. The mechanism of gargling appears to be similar to that of clearing the throat. If the performer feels that gargling is soothing and beneficial, this should be achieved as an 'aphonic' gargle bubbling air through the larynx producing a soft gurgling sound, and avoiding the harsh contact between the arytenoid and vocal folds.

When planning an extensive tour it is wise to anticipate any health problems, and discuss these with one's family physician who knows the performer's past medical history, as well as details of any drug allergies and interactions. Commonly used medications must be carried in hand luggage and not packed in large suitcases which could get lost.

A generic travel kit is essential, particularly if travelling to a new destination. It would be useful for the performer to take simple analgesics which do not contain aspirin, such as paracetamol or acetaminophen. A supply of a suitable antacid to combat any oesophageal reflux should be included, and if it has proved a troublesome problem in the past, a more definitive preparation such as ranitidine or omeprazole should be available. Anti-diarrhoea preparations are worth considering and, if the performer is subject to frequent upper respiratory tract infections, then a 7-day supply of broad spectrum antibiotics should be included.

Nose sprays can be included, but should only be used sparingly if there is persistent nasal stuffiness and the user should be made aware of the likely rebound effect when the medication wears off. Nasal sprays are sometimes useful on flights to prevent middle ear problems in the performer flying with a stuffy nose. Recently developed ear plugs allow for gradual adjustment of pressure during flight, and may be worth consideration. An ephedrine preparation such as Sudafed may be helpful as a decongestant, although it might cause some slight tremor which could be heard in the voice and also causes insomnia and irritability.

Sleeping tablets may help to combat jet lag. The tablets prescribed should be short-acting, and should be without any form of hangover. It is important, as with all drugs, that the performer should not be exposed to a new medication 24 hours before a performance, but should stick to preparations which he has safely tried before.

A few words about vitamins are in order. Many of us take vitamins as a dietary supplement. A great deal has been written about vitamins, and their role in preventing infections, slowing ageing, and generally improving the quality of life. It is important, however, not to overmedicate with vitamins. The fat-soluble vitamins (such as vitamins A, D and E) can accumulate in the body to toxic levels. The water-soluble vitamins (B and C) are not stored, but in mega-doses may (especially vitamin C) act as a diuretic, and thus dry out the vocal tract. Further, vitamin B6 (niacin, nicotinic acid) is a vasodilator, and must be viewed with the same caution as other vasodilators and blood thinners by singers who are prone to vocal fold haemorrhage.

In addition to vitamins, health food stores sell dietary supplements which may be potentially harmful. These are not vitamins, and should not be taken recklessly. Singers should be especially wary of hormone or steroid precursor substances. Some of these, such as pregnenolone and DHEA (dihydroepiandrosterone), are touted as 'anti-ageing' medications, but lack the supervision accorded to other hormones. DHEA specifically may cause some masculinization, including facial hair in women. The effect on the larynx may be similar to other androgenic hormones, causing an irreversible darkening of the voice.

Local anaesthetics may lessen the discomfort of a sore throat. However, they will also interfere with sensation in the larynx and pharynx and the performer will lose the sensation for fine control. Thus, the use of topical local anaesthetic sprays and lozenges in performers is very questionable, and fraught with danger.

Pain is a warning sign in the throat, and the sensation is dulled by topical anaesthesia. If anaesthetics and analgesics are needed to help the performer continue, then further injury, possibly severe, will be inevitable.

Alcohol, barbiturates, sedatives, hypnotics and marijuana, although appearing to have a calming effect, blunt sensation for a good performance and depression follows. Instrumental musicians have found Beta blocker drugs helpful in quelling anxiety and reducing the fine tremor in string players. However, although these drugs may have a place in patients with excessive stage fright, they are contraindicated in asthmatics and can on occasion produce fatigue, depression and impotence. This subject is also dealt with in the chapter on anxiety. Voice professionals who take these drugs may well feel that they have given a splendid rendition, but not infrequently it is a lack-lustre performance. If the performer is extremely anxious and despite counselling decides to resort to a beta blocker, the drug should be tried out on one or two occasions well before the actual performance.

Sedatives must be used with caution, but are sometimes necessary when an over-tired actor or singer is kept awake at night by his anxieties. There is no place for stimulants of the Pep pill variety. A performer influenced by drugs may perceive his voice to be outstanding at the very moment that the sound heard by the audience may be lacking in quality and fine control. Many performers in the West End of London habitually gargle and swallow port before going on stage. Alcohol acts as a muscle relaxant and depressant, much like a tranquillizer and control of the vocal folds and sensitivity of the throat are likely to be impaired. The alcohol is only giving the performer a false sense of security. In addition, alcohol has a drying effect on the tissues of the vocal tract and in the course of time, especially with spirits (hard liquor), there is a resultant chronic irritation. The persistent hoarse or raspy voice is the hallmark of a chronic drinker. The performer who resorts to drugs develops a more tolerant judgement of his own performance and he has a lower critical appraisal of his work at a time when these faculties should be at their sharpest. The singer's or actor's performance is more reliable when he can use his own inner resources, confidence and technique, to allow emotions to flow freely.

11

General medical considerations in the vocal performer

Reflux laryngitis

Sometimes a professional voice user whose history is non-specific will seek advice. There may be little in his description of symptoms which indicates any particular diagnosis at the time. However, he may complain of a foul taste in the mouth in the mornings on rising, the necessity for prolonged warm-up time, and an unexplained non-productive cough. Other less common symptoms may be elicited such as wheezing, asthmatic tendencies and non-cardiac chest pain which may be substernal or retrosternal. There may be an awareness of a bitter, acid taste in the mouth, halitosis and sometimes a history of heartburn. These symptoms are suggestive of the laryngopharyngeal manifestations of gastro-oesophageal reflux. There may also be a history of a sensation of a lump in the throat, or that something has caught in the lower part of the throat itself. As a result, the patient frequently keeps clearing his throat and there may be episodes of laryngeal spasm accompanied by the coughing in the middle of the night. Not infrequently a professional voice user may complain of a post-nasal drip, although examination of the nose and X-rays of the sinuses are unremarkable. These performers not infrequently receive topical sprays, antihistamines and antibiotics and even surgery for the so-called post-nasal drip, but many of the symptoms mentioned may well be caused or aggravated by reflux problems.

Laryngopharyngeal reflux is quite common among singers and actors. The stress of performance not infrequently stimulates acid secretion and the performance itself requires markedly increased abdominal pressure, which works against the oesophageal sphincter. As a full stomach interferes with abdominal support, many singers and actors perform without eating but tend to consume large meals late in the evening and retire to bed soon afterwards. This increases the tendency to develop reflux laryngitis.

The findings of laryngopharyngeal reflux vary, but classically they include markedly reddened arytenoids, with the redness extending along the posterior third of the vocal folds. In more chronic and severe cases, marked swelling, granulomas (Plate 14) and contact ulceration may be present in the posterior part of the larynx. Not infrequently the obvious finding is diffuse swelling with less obvious redness and this oedema can create the illusion of 'sulcus vocalis' as a result of swelling in the subglottic area.

In the general management of this condition, it is important that, where appropriate, the patient should lose weight, stop smoking and avoid alcohol and also meals with high fat contents. The head of the bed should be propped up by 15 to 30 cm and the performer should avoid eating large meals within 3 hours of retiring. This may be difficult for singers and actors, but it is wiser for them to eat larger meals at breakfast and lunchtime and settle for a very light evening meal. Patients should avoid citric juices, tomatoes and tomato-based products, coffee, onions, chocolates, cola drinks, beer, milk, chewing gum, breath fresheners, cough drops and peppermints. These tend to increase acid production and do not provide neutralization. Large quantities of vitamin C (ascorbic acid) may also aggravate these symptoms and drugs that lower oesophageal sphincter pressure should be excluded. Antihistamines and non-steroidal anti-inflammatory drugs (NSAIDs) should be avoided for they may markedly worsen mucosal damage in patients with severe oesophagitis.

Patients with reflux problems should avoid stooping, jogging and press-ups. Patients should be prescribed antacids or an antacid alginate compound to take at times that are most likely to provoke symptomatic reflux, i.e. after meals and at bedtime. If symptoms persist then acid reducing drugs such as ranitidine or the more effective anti-secretor drug omeprazole, should be prescribed on a trial basis. This latter drug will, in the vast majority of patients, get rid of the symptoms and heal any erosive oesophagitis within 4 weeks. However, in many patients treatment will have to continue for 4–6 months together with the general antireflux measures. Patients also have to be treated in addition with another class of agents (prokinetic drugs) which increase lower oesophageal pressure thereby reducing the number of reflux episodes and consequently the total duration of oesophageal exposure to corrosive stomach contents. Among these, cisapride has proved useful. A small group of patients who are not controlled successfully with medical measures can undergo very successful laparoscopic fundoplication surgery for gastro-oesophageal reflux disease, achieving long-term relief of reflux symptoms in 90% of patients.

Performers with posterior laryngitis and granulomas may benefit from voice therapy in addition to the antireflux measures discussed. The greater vigour and longer approximation of the arytenoid cartilages during low register speech produces angulation of the arytenoids and exposure of the contacting surface to scraping injuries. High-speed photography has demonstrated clearly that the loudness of a forceful attack (coup de glotte) during explosive phonation can easily result in injury to the delicate structures of the arytenoid process. Treatment by a voice therapist is aimed to raise the pitch and stop throat clearing and, as mentioned above, the physician should treat any acid reflux problems. Contact granulomas and ulcers occur more frequently in tense, hard-driving people. These individuals sometimes abuse their voices by excessive speaking, often intentionally producing a low pitch, 'macho' voice, currently popular with professional broadcasters. This group tend to be late eaters, heavy drinkers, banquet attenders and speakers. It is now generally accepted that the common mechanism in all cases of contact ulcers and granulomas of the larynx is trauma. Repeated coughing with a chest infection or throat clearing initiated either by acid regurgitation or the presence of thick mucus on the vocal folds and misuse of the voice are precipitating factors.

If a patient tends to be underweight and complies strictly with the treatment recommendation and does not show improvement within a month, then there may be a more significant gastrointestinal dysfunction or the diagnosis is incorrect. Bulimia should be suspected in the differential diagnosis, but difficulty arises in the rare situation where patients deny the fear of becoming fat or disturbance of body image. The constant self-induced vomiting can cause dental erosion with poor gum hygiene.

Allergy

Allergies can affect the nose, the throat and the lower tracheobronchial tree. These symptoms can vary from mild irritation to troublesome sneezing, nasal obstruction, an irritant throat and bronchospasm. The term hay fever is a misnomer, for it is not caused by hay, and secondly does not produce fever. However, it can produce a blocked, runny and itchy nose and eyes with bouts of sneezing, irritation of the throat, and excessive mucous production in the nose and throat. It is caused by allergy to airborne particles that are inhaled. Summer colds are not colds in the usual sense of the word, for they are not due to virus infections. Instead they are, like hay fever, allergies to certain airborne particles. Like hay fever, summer colds are common terms for the medical condition known as allergic rhinitis. It has been estimated that more that 14 million Americans suffer from allergic rhinitis; for some it is a mere nuisance, and for others it is markedly debilitating.

When a plant or animal substance which is foreign to the human, invades the body through the membranes of the nose, throat or eyes, an immune reaction occurs which is intended to counteract such invasion. Under ordinary circumstances, this is a helpful and natural protection. Nevertheless, some individuals exhibit an exaggerated inflammatory response to certain substances which are termed allergens. These allergic patients tend to have a family history of this problem. Allergens stimulate the body to form sensitizing antibodies which then combine with the allergens and this combination causes the body to release a number of chemicals that produce undesirable effects. Histamine is the best known of these chemicals, for it causes swelling of the nasal membrane (rhinitis), itching, irritations and excessive mucous production. Other patients are allergic to moulds, which are fungi and are widespread in nature. They spoil bread, rot fruit and grow on dead leaves, grass, hay and straw. The mould allergy season is long and mould spores may be in the air all year round, except when snow covers the ground. Indoor moulds grow on house plants and in their soil, but they also occur in damp places such as basements, laundry rooms and humidifiers. Moulds can also be found in cheeses and fermented alcohol products.

Patients may also be allergic to cats, dogs, horses and other pets, wool and feathers and house dust. House dust is a complex mixture of disintegrated cellulose (furniture stuffing), moulds, danders, i.e. from household animals and insect parts and small mites.

In the general management of troublesome allergies, it is wise to change air filters monthly in heating and air conditioning systems or install an air purifier. Windows and doors should be closed during the heavy pollinating season and plants and animals that are suspect of carrying mildew should be banned from reception and living room areas. Feather pillows, woollen blankets and woollen clothing should be changed to cotton or synthetic materials and mattresses and pillows should be enclosed in plastic (barrier) cloth or material impervious to the house dust mite.

If the performer has a short period of seasonal allergy and is able to control the symptoms well with mild antihistamines which do not have any marked drying effect, then provided the artist is well versed with the medication and its properties he should be allowed to use it when necessary. However, there may not be any ideal preparation and the performer may well have to experiment with several antihistamines when he is 'resting' before finding a medication which largely abolishes the main symptoms. Although food allergies can occasionally play a part, and their identification can usually be determined by an exclusion diet, the main problems for performers are usually related to pollens, animal dander, moulds and dust. The international performer will cross many times zones and pollination bands. Thus the allergen can be more problematical in certain areas of the globe, and indeed in certain regions of the same country.

Older theatres and concert halls because of their numerous curtains, backstage drapes and somewhat antiquated dressing room facilities that are not always thoroughly cleaned, can cause allergic symptoms due to dust and accumulated mould. These institutions have floors and boards which have not been vacuumed since the day that they were nailed down. As a result nasal obstruction and conjunctivitis may develop, due to a generalized irritation of the mucosal lining of the eye and respiratory tract. The nose, apart from its function as the organ of smell, warms and also humidifies the air en route to the lungs. Nasal obstruction can result in a drying effect on the pharynx and larynx as a result of mouth breathing, and this will affect the quality of mucosal secretion, causing decreased lubrication and the sensation of a tickling cough and an irritated throat.

Sometimes in a very noxious, dusty environment backstage, a filtering mask such as is used by tradespeople in dust-laden industrial sites, or a surgical mask that does not contain fibreglass, can be helpful.

If the symptoms are troublesome then further investigation can be carried out by skin testing or by taking a sample of the patient's blood and measuring the immunoglobulin (IgE) antibody response to various allergens being tested. Treatment ideally consists of avoiding the noxious irritant, taking various suppressive medications, and desensitizations. The membranes of the nose have an abundant supply of arteries, veins and capillaries which have a great capacity for both expansion and constriction. Normally these blood vessels are in a half constricted, half opened state, but when a person exercises vigorously his hormone stimulation (adrenaline) increases. The adrenaline causes constriction or squeezing of the nasal blood vessels which shrinks the nasal membrane so that the air passage is opened up and the person breathes more freely. The opposite takes place when an allergic attack or cold develops. The blood vessels expand, and the membranes become engorged (full of excess blood) and the nose becomes stuffy and blocked. In addition to allergies and infection, other events can cause nasal blood vessels to expand, leading to vasomotor rhinitis. These include psychological stress, inadequate thyroid function, pregnancy, certain drugs given to lower blood pressure and overuse or prolonged use of decongestive nasal sprays. In the early stages of each of these disorders the nasal stuffiness is temporary and reversible. However, if the condition persists long enough, the blood vessels lose their capacity to constrict and they become somewhat like varicose veins. The vessels fill up when the patient lies down and when he lies on his side, the lower side becomes congested. The congestion often interferes with sleep and so it is helpful for the patient with a stuffy nose to sleep with the head of the bed elevated 10 cm (4 inches). Surgery can, on occasions, offer dramatic and long-term relief in this problem, but has little part to play in the truly allergic nose.

Certain nasal sprays containing topical steroids such as beclomethasone dipropionate (Beconase) or budesonide (Rhinocort) may be helpful in order to decrease the swelling of the nasal mucosa. However, it must be realized that these preparations take a few days to begin working and should be used at the minimum therapeutic dose. Even though they act locally on the nose, very occasionally they can cause fungal infection of the pharynx and vocal fold, but this is more prevalent in debilitated individuals. They can also, sometimes, cause very slight nose bleeds.

Decongestant tablets may be useful, but it must be remembered that many compounds containing pseudoephedrine can, if taken late at night, act as a stimulus and prevent normal sleep and in the older male group are likely to cause some urinary symptoms.

Asthma and respiratory dysfunction

Mild, obstructive lung disease can impair the performer's 'support' and result in increased muscle tension in the neck and tongue and resulting abusive voice technique producing vocal nodules. Occasionally this is brought to light in a student who has to sing or speak when doing dance and movement classes, and becomes somewhat wheezy as a result of exertion at the end of the session. This exercise-induced asthma may not be easy to determine, and occasionally may also develop when an artist is somewhat late for his performance and rushes to the theatre on a cold evening and becomes wheezy on arrival. The vocal artist with subclinical asthma may also have this triggered by anxiety. Although he may well have normal pulmonary function at the beginning of the performance, supporting well and singing with a good technique, as the evening continues the pulmonary function decreases, impairing support. This results in upper thoracic breathing and leads on to adopting abusive vocal techniques. The performer who has asthmatic tendencies should undergo pulmonary function tests with a chest physician sympathetic to his problems and who is aware that certain inhalers can be somewhat irritant to the larynx and vasodilator drugs might cause a mild tremor which can be audible during soft singing.

Although the effects of inhaled corticosteroids on the smooth muscle of the vocal folds is unclear, vocal dysfunction due to fungal deposits can occur with long-term exposure (Plate 15). Very occasionally a decrease in lower oesophageal sphincter tone can occur with oral bronchodilators, and increase the likelihood of aggravating gastro-oesophageal reflux symptoms. Sometimes a chronic cough may be the only symptom of asthma and the fully fledged presentation of wheezy respiration with chest tightness may not be initially apparent.

Exercise-induced asthma is a well-known entity, and is largely due to changes in the airway tone produced by the hyperventilation. Susceptible subjects hurrying to their evening performance in cold, dry air may develop bronchospasm. However, the same group of patients, if they inhale fully saturated air, warmed to 37°C do not have any problem with their air flow.

When any factors are introduced to change adversely breath support, accessory muscles in the head and neck are brought into action. This resulting inappropriate muscle use causes vocal fatigue, decreased control (especially during soft speech), loss of range and other vocal problems. During rigorous physical demands of singing or acting, even slight changes in breath support may produce such problems. Professional actors and singers are particularly attuned to subtle changes in airflow and pressure and because of their vocal demands even slight changes in physical ability may be immediately apparent and potentially disabling.

Obesity and diet

Most actors and singers are extrovert characters, for they would not embark on a career on the stage if they were wholly introspective in nature. Many enjoy living life to the full and enjoy good food and wine. Consequently many well-known performers today and in the past had been markedly overweight and there has grown up a folklore that to be an outstanding opera singer being overweight is a distinct vocal advantage. Singing and acting involves vocal athletics and a fit body and mind is essential to achieve expertise in the field. Good abdominal support, excellent respiratory function and reserve, physical strength and mental and physical endurance are essential to a successful career and vocal longevity. When obesity becomes gross it is associated with well-recognized medical problems. Hypertension occurs far more frequently in overweight people as does an elevated level of cholesterol and an increased incidence of heart disease. Diabetes, especially in the older age group is associated with obesity, as is gastro-oesophageal reflux, varicose veins and hernias. Markedly overweight patients develop respiratory problems as they cannot expand their chest as well as a thinner person and arthritis, especially in the knee joints, develops. Generally, obese individuals are a greater anaesthetic risk during surgery and on the whole have a shorter working life. Overweight people not infrequently snore loudly and may suffer from sleep apnoea and hence may become extremely tired in the afternoon and drop off to sleep when not in bed. Frequently they get depressed because of their weight problem.

In general, obesity can be treated by reduction of calorie intake or increase of calorie expenditure, or both. Although there have been many suggestions that the macronutrient composition of the calorically restricted diet is important for successful weight reduction, there is no firm evidence that a calorie is anything more than a calorie, regardless of the food source from which it has derived, despite the popularity of many calorifically unbalanced 'fad' diets. In principle, it is clear that the aim of weight reduction diet should be to keep normal body composition as well as to attain normal weight. There is no evidence to support the superiority of any form of low calorie diet over that of another. The most common method for promoting calorie expenditure in obese individuals is increased exercise. This results in a significant reduction in the percentage of body fat with a proportional increase in lean body mass. Gradual weight reduction is recommended for people who are obese and dieting should be slow and gradual. The aim should be to lose between 1–1.3 kg (2–3 pounds) per week. Rapid weight loss should be avoided because this can cause minor metabolic disturbances and sometimes a sensation of weakness with resultant changes in vocal quality and endurance. However, the advice of a dietitian should be sought if progress is not made and appetite suppressant drugs only used if absolutely necessary and then, only under strict medical supervision.

Nuts and spicy foods such as chillies and curries should be avoided for not only can they stimulate bouts of coughing and throat clearing but they also can be gastric irritants.

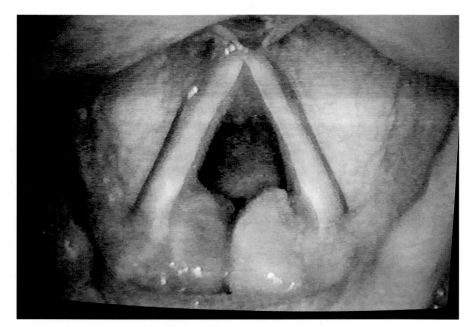

Plate 14 Granulomas

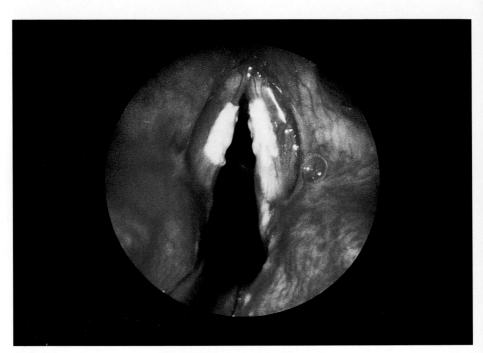

Plate 15 Fungal laryngitis

Halitosis

A degree of halitosis (oral malodour or foetor oris) is common in healthy people, particularly after sleep. For performers who have to work face to face with other people, bad breath or halitosis is a worrying embarrassment. Occasionally neuroses develop over the problem of halitosis and there are many people who compulsively use mouth sprays, mints, mouth fresheners, frequent mouth washes and brush their teeth excessively. Halitosis at other times is a distressing complaint from which few people escape completely and which is still not completely understood. The true prevalence is not known, but one recent study suggested that nearly half of a group of young women (dental hygienists) believed that they sometimes had halitosis. Halitosis may also be imaginary (dilusional halitosis) or a hallucinatory feature in schizophrenia.

Patients who refrain from cleaning their mouths soon develop halitosis, but any form of oral sepsis can produce appreciable malodour, the most common condition being inflammatory plaque-related gingival disease (gingivitis) or periodontal disease (periodontitis). The amount of volatile sulphur compounds and the ratio of methylmercaptan to sulphide are higher in the mouth air from patients with periodontal disease than in that from people with healthy mouths.

Generally, in the morning, the breath is pungent and often disagreeable, which is probably due to the near total cessation of salivary flow during sleep and the accumulation and putrefaction of oral debris, food and saliva. Eating or cleansing the mouth in the morning typically clears bad breath relating from the oral cavity. However, it may not change other factors such as the result of overindulgence of alcohol the previous night, mouth breathing or smoking. Halitosis in the morning may also be related to certain foods eaten the night before, particularly onions, garlic and curries. The odour of morning breath has been shown to occur from the breakdown of cellular proteins and amino acids to odorous, volatile, sulphur-containing compounds such as hydrogen sulphide and methymercaptan. Normal saliva usually is slightly acidic and this suppresses the growth and proliferation of certain bacteria. Saliva removed from the mouth and incubated, quickly becomes alkaline and exceedingly objectionable.

Patients with acid reflux not infrequently complain of a bad odour and an acid taste in the mouth. An empty stomach can also contribute to the creation of an objectionable odour and this may be then noticeable in patients who miss meals and the odour may disappear soon after eating. The source of the hunger breath is uncertain but appears to emanate from the lungs. Even moderate dehydration will lead to decreased salivary flow, favour oral putrefaction of food or epithelial debris and can be corrected easily. Dehydration of the mouth may not only be due to a poor fluid intake, but to chronic mouth breathing and drugs such as antihistamines and diuretics.

Virtually any condition leading to the growth of anaerobic microorganisms will produce an unpleasant smell. Such examples are acute or chronic sinusitis or pharyngitis due to the destruction of the normal physiological mucus blanket of the nose by inflammatory states. The nasal lining that is damaged by the overuse and abuse of nasal drops and sprays can result in a chronic problem – rhinitis medicamentosa. This results in permanent damage to the nasal lining and these people not frequently have a malodour emulating from the nasal cavity.

Chronic infection within tonsils or adenoidal crypts can also be a source of problems, for food and desquamated epithelium trapped within this moist, warm space, form an ideal medium for bacterial growth. This condition can sometimes be helped by cleaning the tonsillar crypts by the use of a water pick or laser cryptolysis.

The management of halitosis requires establishing the presence of true halitosis and assessing its severity. The history and examination should be directed towards eliminating any dietary and systemic causes. A full assessment of oral and dental health is always indicated and, although a dental practitioner is the best trained for this, a periodontologist has a special skill in disorders affecting the gingiva and peridontium.

The most reliable management is to reduce oral flora, particularly anaerobes; this is best achieved by improving oral hygiene by brushing the teeth, cleaning between the teeth, and other means. A simple, inexpensive and effective treatment is to use a mouth rinse of 0.2% aqueous chlorhexidine gluconate, which is remarkably active against a range of organisms in dental plaque and can also reduce halitosis whether judged subjectively or by decreases in volatile sulphides in the mouth air. If the problem is an infection in the nose, pharynx or sinuses, appropriate advice should be sought and halitosis resulting from gastric reflux can be improved substantially by the use of antacids and by the methods outlined in the section on this subject.

Bad breath associated with malabsorption may be improved with dietary changes, an increase in the ingestion of fruits and vegetables and a decrease in dietary fat intake. It is obviously important to make sure that salivary flow is copious. Many masking substances are available commercially, but oil of peppermint follows the same metabolic route as garlic and is of some help. Coffee, strong tea and cola drinks not only increase general nervousness and irritability but can cause a diuresis and relative dehydration. These beverages can also cause an element of gastric irritation, increasing the tendency to aggravate gastro-oesophageal reflux and this can be reflected in frequent throat clearing and vocal fatigue in some people. Herbal teas taken in moderation are said to have some beneficial effect for they may act to thin secretions.

Hiccup

Hiccup is an involuntary quick inspiration interrupted by a quick closure of the vocal folds. Its aetiology is unknown but it is usually benign and of short duration and stops spontaneously or as a result of various self-administrated respiratory manoeuvres. It is often associated with gastric distension, sudden changes in temperature, emotion, or ingestion of alcohol. Hiccups are virtually always self-limiting, but if they occur for longer than 24 hours then further investigations to rule out an underlying disease may have to be carried out. The condition may be inhibited by sipping ice-cold water, gargling or stimulating the outer ear canal. Chlorpromazine may also have a place in treating this condition.

Temporomandibular disorders

Singers appear to be more susceptible to difficulties in the temporomandibular joint (TMJ) than the general population for vocal artists open their mouths widely and repeatedly for long periods of time. Singing often extends the jaw beyond the normal range of motion. The rise of temporomandibular disorders (TMD) among vocalists may be directly related to the singing technique itself. Many jaw problems result from concepts the singer has about arranging ideal resonator space. Hanging the jaw too wide to get resonance may be a reason for TMD symptoms among vocalists. It may be that emphasizing the lateral/circular loose movements of the jaw provides a far more efficient solution to jaw tension than does giving instructions to students to open the mouth as widely as possible. Many singers who have complained of TMD syndrome discover that they no longer have the problem when they learn that they need not hang the jaw in the hope of 'opening the throat'. Muscle tension caused by performance stress is also an aggravating factor.

Singers seeking treatment for TMD nearly always exhibit a greater range of mandibular opening than do non-vocalists with TMD. This condition can result in a decreased range, vocal fatigue, change in the quality or placement of a voice and excess tongue/muscle activity. Painful catching or locking of the TMJ in a wide open mouth position interferes with singing and is often associated with temporal headaches.

If TMD is suspected and the symptoms prove troublesome, professional help is necessary. If a dental problem is suspected to be the cause, then the dentist may be able to assist with splint therapy (used to adjust the bite), night guards (used to stop bruxism and clenching), crowns and medications. An orthodontist opinion should be sought if occlusion problems exist. In severe cases of jaw mis-alignment an oral and maxillofacial surgeon may be needed to correct the TMJ and or jaws. Many hospitals have TMJ clinics with staff who provide a wide range of care.

Hormonal changes and voice

Vocal symptoms associated with the premenstrual phase of the menstrual cycle include a loss of high tones, vocal instability and fatigue, decreased vocal efficiency, uncertainty of pitch and huskiness, together with reduced vocal power and flexibility. This is often more apparent to the singer than the listener. This perceived vocal change is associated with the physiological change in hormone level which results in a drop in oestrogen levels on or about day 21 in the menstrual cycle. As oestrogen levels drop, laryngeal tissues begin to absorb water, causing vocal cord swelling, engorged blood vessels and increased vocal fold mass.

Any change in overall size and mass of the vocal folds is likely to produce some change in vibratory characteristics of the vocal fold with resulting changes as listed above. Submucosal haemorrhages in the vocal folds are not uncommon at this time of the month.

Premenstrual abdominal cramping or bloating is not an infrequent general complaint in the premenstrual phase and since female singers rely to a major degree on abdominal muscle strength for support, this symptom can be troublesome. Performers who are plagued by troublesome premenstrual tension and who are aware of some difficulty in producing high notes should, in order to avoid potential damage to the vocal folds or establishing incorrect vocal habits, minimize rehearsing and attempt to avoid new repertoires or new techniques when the symptoms are most severe. When oral contraceptives are used the voice should be carefully monitored for, in a very small number of women, the 'pill' can adversely alter vocal range and vocal character even after a few months of treatment. If a woman has an extremely important performance and knows that she is normally severely affected by the side-effects of menstruation then it is possible to alter the time of the monthly period by giving an oral contraceptive, but this decision must not be taken lightly.

Menopause occurs in women in their late forties and early fifties and represents the permanent cessation of cyclical menstruation due to a loss of ovarian activity. The production of female hormones is reduced, with blood levels of both oestradiol and progesterone falling to almost undetectable levels. The postmenopausal ovary then secretes androgen (the male hormones) which together with androgens originating from the adrenal glands, leads to a relative excess of the male hormones in the blood stream. Menopause is sometimes associated with general symptoms of insomnia and sleep deprivation as well as hot flushes and psychological changes, genital atrophy together with laryngeal mucosal changes. Cardiovascular disease is more common after the menopause as is osteoporosis and decreased libido.

It should be kept in mind that cessation of menstrual periods is often a late sign of the menopause, and other manifestations may occur earlier.

After the menopause, voices typically drop in fundamental frequencies due to the marked reduction or cessation of oestrogen but the continuing production of androgen. Women near the menopause or in the menopause also have to deal with age-related factors apart from hormonal changes. These may include atrophy of laryngeal muscle and vocal fold thickening, stiffening of the laryngeal cartilages and a decrease in lung power. Around the menopause therefore, the singer may notice breathiness, a decrease in overall vocal range, especially the upper register. There may be development of a tremolo, decreased breath control, vocal fatigue and pitch inaccuracies, together with a change in the characteristics of the vibrato.

Occasionally, low oestrogen voice changes may precede the interruption of menses and it is sometimes desirable to introduce oestrogen replacement even before menstrual periods become irregular or stop. As with any medication used by a performer, hormone replacement therapy must be used with caution and it has to be individually tailored. Women with career demands on their voice should be offered menopausal hormonal therapy and appropriate medical supervision by doctors who really understand the stresses and strains of the acting and singing professions. For women who have a spontaneous menopause (not surgically induced), and still have the uterus, oestrogen treatment has to be combined with progesterone in order to prevent adverse affects from long-term unopposed oestrogen on the endometrium of the uterus. Progesterones are applied sequentially (for 12 days every month) or continuously and various combined menopausal regimens contain different types of progesterone. While it is assumed that oestrogens reverse adverse changes in the female voice occurring at the menopause, there is distinct uncertainty concerning the effects of progesterones on the voice and some types of progesterones even have an adverse effect. Some menopausal regimens contain progesterones with relatively high androgenic properties and this leads to masculinization of the voice, causing deepening and lowering of the fundamental frequency and changes in timbre.

Oestrogen replacement therapy also gives women a sense of well-being and many have used this therapy for decades without obvious complications. In the short term HRT may cause un-wanted side-effects (such as breast swelling and, in women taking a progestogen, persistent symptoms akin to premenstrual syndrome). For as long as it is taken, HRT seems to increase the risk of thromboembolism. If used for longer than 10 years it increases the risk of breast cancer. With careful selection of the HRT regimen used, the unwanted effects can be minimized. Ultimately, however, it is for the woman to decide if the advantages outweigh the potential risks. The matter should be fully discussed with the patient's endocrinologist and gynaecologist.

Oestrone, a relatively weak oestrogen, is one female hormone little affected by the loss of ovarian function. It is produced almost exclusively from androgens through conversion in fatty (adipose) tissue. Thus, oestrone becomes the major circulating oestrogen after the menopause. The fact that oestrone is produced in fat tissue might explain why some markedly overweight singers are less affected by menopausal changes.

Post-menopausal women who experience vocal difficulties due to the ageing process can reverse some of these effects through voice therapy and regular vocal training and general physical exercise. Regular vocal training often eliminates the tremolo and improves agility, pitch accuracy and reduces vocal fatigue. Singers in the post-menopausal phase learn to compensate for physiological changes due to hormonal changes such as vocal fold oedema. These compensatory tactics are sometimes vocally abusive and can lead to long-term vocal problems. It is suggested that women experiencing vocal difficulties secondary to menopausal changes obtain the help of a singing voice specialist/therapist and a laryngologist who specializes in working with singers who can rule out any vocal fold pathology and, with his team, eliminate any vocally abusive compensatory techniques.

Androgens, which are commonly used for endometriosis, are most certainly contraindicated in female singers for they cause unsteadiness of the voice, lowering of fundamental voice frequency and rapid changes in timbre. When therapy is stopped the voice improves but the pre-treatment high tones rarely return, although the lower tones can be fuller than before the androgen therapy was commenced.

Changes similar to premenstrual symptoms occur in pregnancy and subtle vocal changes are often perceived by the patient. In addition, in mid and late pregnancy important changes occur in abdominal support, associated with distension during pregnancy which interferes with abdominal muscle function and also an altered centre of gravity.

On rare occasions, a deepening of the voice can occur in male and female performers due to hypothyroidism. Vocal fatigue, hoarseness, muffling, loss of range, an increase in weight and a feeling of a lump in the throat may be present even with mild deficiency of the thyroid hormone. The typical patient dislikes cold weather, becomes lethargic and on laryngeal examination, the vocal folds are swollen. Thyroid replacement therapy is very effective in reversing many of the changes, but periodic monitoring of thyroid hormone levels by an endrocrinologist is essential.

Anabolic steroids which are related to male hormones, in addition to their other hazards may alter the voice, causing a deepening and coarseness of the voice as a result of some masculization changes which are usually not reversible.

A visit to the laryngologist

Every singer or actor will, at some time in his or her career, visit a laryngologist. Unlike most other patients, vocal performers bring their livelihood to the physician, and need specific advice and treatment, often on an emergency basis. In order to make the most of this consultation, the performer must know what to expect, and how to make use of the advice given.

What to look for in a laryngologist

Most ear, nose and throat specialists treat voice patients. There are, however, those who have taken a special interest in the voice and the performer. This special interest often includes a personal interest in music, as a singer, instrumentalist or avid listener. Further, it entails the acquisition of additional expertise regarding the voice. Since voice problems are generally not taught during resident training, these physicians may have taken additional training, observed other laryngologists, or have acquired insight over years of working with singers, voice teachers or speech therapists. Voice problems have a special vocabulary which includes the musical and psychological, as well as the medical. Dealing with the professional voice requires empathy, insight and often some sacrifice of time and convenience. For every international star, these physicians will treat dozens of impoverished young students, and willingly accept their financial limitations in exchange for the opportunity to advance the cause of music and the vocal arts.

Most vocal performers meet their laryngologist either by referral from colleagues, their agent or theatre management. When on tour, or in a foreign city, these referrals are helpful: treatment is usually short term, and the word-of-mouth recommendation of colleagues is a useful standard. At home, however, singers should take some time in selecting a laryngologist. Since the relationship will likely be a long-term one (although not necessarily involving frequent visits), we suggest that the patient interview or 'audition' several laryngologists. The singer should look for expertise and availability on the laryngologist's part. Of equal importance, however, is the chemistry between physician and patient. A sympathetic and caring physician is attuned to the physical and mental problems a performer may encounter. A comfortable relationship should develop, which will allow the patient to telephone the physician or visit on short notice, should the need arise.

Among laryngologists managing singers, there are two schools of thought. The traditional school relies primarily on medications, reassurance and psychological support. This school is congruent with the non-anatomical, visual imagery type of vocal pedagogy, and has stood the test of time in the context of the traditional physician–patient relationship. There is, however, a newer trend, both in voice teaching and vocal medicine. This school familiarizes the singer with the anatomy and physiology of the singing voice, using photographs and video recordings. The singer knows not only what the voice sounds like, but is equally comfortable looking at the larynx. This approach gives the patient greater insight, which can lead to active involvement in the treatment process. This is exemplified by the use of visual biofeedback to correct posturing abnormalities of the larynx. Although the philosophy and approach of these schools seem divergent, the ultimate aim is the same: to restore the singing voice and optimize its expressive powers. The ideal management of singers therefore should probably be a synthesis of these two schools. Ideally, every singer should know the appearance of her larynx, and have in her possession at least a still photograph of her vocal folds as a base line for comparison. Although the quality of these prints may vary, depending on equipment and illumination, photographs are particularly useful when the singer needs to consult a new physician on tour. Even with the best of intentions, such a physician may misinterpret the appearance of the larynx without the benefit of a 'normal' photograph.

Vocal performers should also be familiar with stroboscopic images of the vibrating vocal folds and, if possible, obtain a video recording of their larynx performing various vocal tasks.

Most larynges have minute and insignificant imperfections, and appreciation of these will relieve much of the performer's anxiety.

In addition, however, there is a time for medications, sprays and injections. A performance that cannot be cancelled, an acute illness, a short but gruelling tour may call for specific treatment which has little to do with the minutiae of anatomy and physiology. The ideal laryngologist is one who has both approaches in his repertoire, and can individualize treatment to the patient and the situation.

The first visit

Once a laryngologist has been found, we recommend a 'baseline' visit. This serves several purposes. It introduces the actor or singer to the physician, and a medical record can be established for consultation later, when advice may be sought by long-distance telephone. It also allows the physician to become familiar with the singer's larynx in its normal state. Photographs or video recordings can be generated, with copies made for both singer and physician. We cannot overly stress the usefulness of serial photodocumentation in following a pathological process, such as a vocal fold haemorrhage.

History

When a singer indicates that he has something wrong with his voice, the laryngologist should take him seriously, for the performer is frightened of losing his livelihood. The way he gives his history should be carefully listened to and his body language observed and the physician should be on the lookout for misusage. Singers frequently have trained the singing voice much better than the speaking voice and this can cause a problem in musical theatre. Here the performer uses the singing voice far more effectively than his speaking voice and this is particularly so if he has to play a part using a dialect or accent that he is unfamiliar with. The physician should watch and listen for clarity and see if there is any breathiness apparent. Breathiness may come from bad technique or it may be from something that is actually intrinsically wrong. Similarly, any other abnormality, heard, seen or otherwise perceived, should be noted.

On the patient's part, the singer should, at the time of initial visit, be prepared to present a full vocal history. This is often done by way of a written questionnaire, but may also be obtained verbally by the physician. The history includes details of the entire singing career, the type of singing, details of training obtained, and repertoire. The laryngologist also needs to know in detail any vocal problems, however trivial, which have developed over the years of singing. Minor but recurrent problems, such as transient hoarseness, may be mistakenly attributed to discrete and unrelated medical conditions, whereas they in fact represent symptoms of a chronic laryngeal problem that never completely resolved. These conditions can only be identified if a temporal sequence of the 'episodes' is clearly presented.

The singer should be able to describe the specific problem, keeping in mind that unless the laryngologist is well versed in vocal terminology, the complaint may need to be demonstrated. Terms such as passaggio, chest voice and falsetto are not taught in medical school: unless the singer can convincingly demonstrate the difficulty experienced, there is a danger that the complaint may appear trivial, and no help will be obtained. In some practices, the patient will be asked to perform specific vocal tasks in order that the difficulties may be uncovered. A keyboard is helpful. Some singers will bring tapes from a performance to illustrate the problem.

During history taking, the physician should gain a full understanding of both the problem and of the vocal tasks the singer must undertake. An amateur choral singer faces challenges different from a rock singer or an operatic performer.

Examination

Proper examination addresses both structure and function. The anatomy of the vocal apparatus is examined through a complete assessment of the head and neck area, including the ears, nose, mouth, pharynx and larynx. Additional areas of potential importance are the chest and the posture, which is in turn affected by the spine and the abdomen. The larynx may be visualized either with a mirror, or by techniques of endoscopy. Each method has its advantages and disadvantages, and will be discussed below. Functional examination may be carried out by the physician, or in conjunction with a voice therapist. A personal background in singing is helpful in putting the patient through a series of vocal tasks. The fundamental pitch of the speaking voice is noted. This is often untrained and too low, therefore potentially more abusive than the actual singing technique. The limits of the singing voice, from low chest to falsetto are assessed, focusing particularly on the passaggio and the top of the voice. The soft voice is especially telling of vocal difficulties, and soft (*pp*) attacks at the top are attempted.

Anatomical and physiological examination come together during laryngeal stroboscopy, and this is also discussed below.

Techniques of laryngoscopy

There are three ways to visualize the larynx in the consulting room: with a mirror, with a flexible laryngoscope and with a rigid laryngoscope. The fourth way, direct examination, involves a larger laryngoscope, and is done under general anaesthesia in the operating room. This is discussed in detail in the section on microsurgery.

Mirror examination involves placing a small dental-type mirror in the back of the mouth. The patient's tongue is pulled forward, opening the back of the throat. The mirror is tilted at an angle, and allows both the beams from the examiner's headlight, as well as his vision, to see around the back of the tongue, and down to the larynx. The examination is simple, rapid and relatively comfortable. It gives an undistorted panoramic view of the hypopharynx and larynx and, depending on colour temperature of the light, produces a clear optical image. Since the examiner uses binocular vision, mirror examination gives the most three-dimensional image of the three techniques described.

Mirror examination also has disadvantages. Patients with a sensitive gag reflex cannot tolerate the placement of the mirror. A topical anaesthetic spray is helpful. If the patient is uncomfortable, the physician may gain only a momentary glimpse of the vocal folds. In patients with a curled or overhanging epiglottis, part of the larynx may be obscured, and the anterior commissure in particular is difficult to visualize. Another shortcoming of mirror examination is that the fleeting image cannot be recorded for review or analysis.

Flexible fibreoptic laryngoscopy involves passing a thin instrument through the nose. The instrument is a flexible cable containing numerous optic bundles. The tip of the endoscope can be bent, and the instrument is easily directed to the back of the throat, and then down to the oro- and hypopharynx. By turning the instrument and adjusting its tip, the entire hypopharynx and larynx may be seen.

One advantage of the flexible endoscope is the minimal discomfort to the patient. The gag reflex is entirely bypassed. The nasal cavity is usually sprayed with an anaesthetic/decongestant, and the instrument passes through smoothly. Another advantage is the ability to look below an obstructing epiglottis, and visualize the full length of the vocal folds. A skillful examiner can advance the endoscope to within millimetres of the surface of the vocal folds. The scope is built so that it produces a panoramic image, pulling in the visual field at its periphery. This compensates for some decrease in manoeuvrability as compared to the mirror.

Some physicians feel that, by not pulling the tongue forward, the anatomical relations in the back of the throat are better seen in their natural position. Abnormal posturing or movements of the supraglottic areas can be observed. The patient can also sing or phonate in relative comfort during fibreoptic examination. This is not possible with the mirror or rigid rod. The flexible laryngoscope may also be attached to a video camera, still camera or stroboscope to capture the image for the record, or subsequent analysis or instruction. The main disadvantage of the flexible scope is the lower quality of the image. The image is transmitted as hundreds of tiny bits (analogous but not identical to pixels) which is 'synthesized' by the examiner's eye. The small black spaces between the image bits degrade the image, and may lead to inadvertent oversight of small lesions, such as a telangiectasis. With repeated use, the fibres may break, and each broken fibre appears as another black dot in the image. The optics of the individual fibreoptic bundle are not as good as the mirror, or the rigid laryngoscope, described below. The flexible scope image also distorts at the periphery, the price paid for a panoramic view. If the image is recorded, it is usually small, and there is further loss of definition with magnification.

The rigid (transoral) laryngoscope is a chrome-plated metal tube which is placed into the mouth. The end of the scope is angled (usually 70° or 90°). The patient opens her mouth, and the tongue is again held forward. When placed in the mouth, the end of the scope extends into the oropharynx. It then 'looks around the corner', like a periscope, and looks at the hypopharynx and larynx. The laryngoscope contains a series of lenses which transmit and focus the image. The comfort level of this examination is similar to that of the mirror, and most patients are able to cooperate sufficiently.

Of all three techniques, rigid laryngoscopy gives the overall best optic image of the larynx (Plate 16). While not a true reflected image, like the mirror, the image passes through a series of air lenses which are optically superior to the flexible fibre. The image is magnified, and is usually transmitted to a video recorder for further magnification. This is the preferred technique for video stroboscopy, since the free margins of the vocal folds are clearly seen. The image is usually recorded for easy retrieval. There are only two disadvantages to this technique. Some patients are unable to tolerate the instrument, even with instruction and practice, a situation which never occurs with the flexible endoscope. Patients with short chins, large tongues and shallow pharynges are particularly difficult. An overhanging epiglottis may present a persistent visual obstacle. Secondly, patients cannot freely demonstrate full vocal function, since the tongue, and attached hyoid complex, are pulled forward.

Rigid endoscopy gives a superior image of the larynx, but its insertion again involves some anatomical distortion of the base of tongue and hypopharynx. Overall, however, rigid endoscopy is the preferred method for examining and recording the appearance of the vocal folds in their fine anatomical detail.

Laryngeal stroboscopy

1 Principle of stroboscopy

Visual images tend to persist on the retina. A series of individual images are 'connected' by this tendency to persist, and give the illusion of smooth continuous movement. This is the principle by which projected film, a series of static images, produces an illusion of movement on the screen.

Stroboscopic lighting produces a series of rapid light bursts. By illuminating moving objects, the viewer's eye is given a series of static images, which are subjectively connected, each one to the next. If the images differ only slightly (slow rate of motion, or rapid rate of flashes), the movement appears smooth. If the images differ significantly (rate of movement significantly faster than rate of flashes), the movement appears jerky and jagged. This is the effect seen at discotheques or rock concerts.

If the movement is repetitive, it has a frequency, the number of times per second that the movement occurs. If the stroboscopic flashes are synchronized to occur at the same frequency as the movement, the moving object will be illuminated at the same instant. The images will show the object at the same point in its repetitive movement, and it will therefore appear not to be moving. This technique is used in industry to examine rapidly moving machines for wear. If the rate of movement and the flashes of light occur at slightly different rates, the movement will be illuminated at a different point in its cycle, creating the visual illusion of slow motion.

2 Laryngeal application

Laryngeal strobosocopy uses exactly this principle. For example, the vocal folds vibrate at 1000 cycles per second (around B above middle C), and their vibration triggers the strobe light generator. If the light falls at the beginning of each cycle, the vocal folds appear still, and closed (adducted). If the light, still synchronized, flashes in mid-cycle, the folds appear open. By slightly shifting the moment of the flash, the glottis can be 'frozen' at any moment of its vibratory cycle.

If the glottic vibrations and the strobe are at slightly different rates, the light will illuminate a different moment in each sub-sequent cycle, and create an illusion of slow motion. This is particularly useful to the examiner, as it allows him to see how the folds open and close. In laryngeal stroboscopy, the light generator can be attached to either a flexible fibreoptic laryngo-scope, or the transoral rigid laryngoscope. There is no other

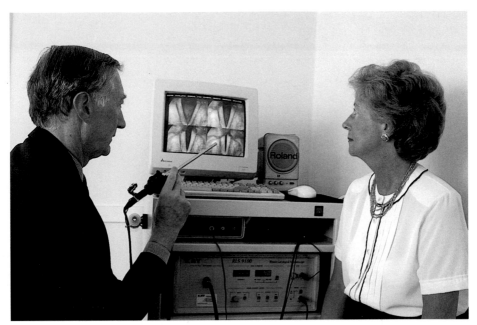

Plate 16 Rigid laryngoscope

technique (apart from ultra-high speed cinematography, expensive, cumbersome and not practical), to slow down the vocal folds in this way.

What does stroboscopy reveal? The vibration of the vocal folds is a complex series of movements, which varies greatly with frequency and intensity. Normally the vibration is confined mostly to the mucosa covering the folds. This mucosa, attached loosely to the underlying vocal ligament and muscle, seems to flow in a series of waves, along the surface of the vocal fold. Different degrees of vibration are seen in chest, head or falsetto voice.

Stroboscopy is an essential part of a complete laryngeal examination. It need not be performed every time the patient is seen, but it reveals aspects of anatomy and function that are not seen by any other technique. For example, mild degrees of oedema (swelling), may not be seen by static examination but will manifest as stiffness with loss of the mucosal wave during stroboscopy. Unlike a blood test, stroboscopy is very technique-dependent. How it is performed and how it is analysed varies greatly from one examiner to another.

Discussion

Once the examination is complete, the laryngologist will discuss his findings with the patient. Anatomy drawings or models are helpful. Video or still photographs bring the problem home to the patient. There should be an opportunity for the singer to ask questions or raise concerns. If there are questions relating to repertoire or vocal technique, it is helpful to have an experienced voice therapist available to complete the discussion.

Treatment

As a treatment plan is formulated, the patient should again feel that she is part of the decision-making process. Most chronic vocal problems have three components: anatomical, functional (physiological) and psychological. While medication may be effective for the anatomical problem, to change effectively patterns of misuse and to recognize and address psychological problems requires that the patient be an equal partner in the treatment plan. Of course, for acute or minor complaints, medication alone is adequate, and does not require such extensive analysis. The importance of distinguishing truly acute problems from chronic problems with acute exacerbations cannot therefore be underestimated.

Follow-up visits

Subsequent visits may vary in length and complexity. Once a solid base-line has been established at the initial visit, follow-up visits may consist of briefer examinations to monitor a polyp or haemorrhage, without the time and expense of videolaryngoscopy. Once singer and laryngologist have established a good working relationship, even a transatlantic telephone call can be therapeutic.

13

Surgery and the vocal artist

It is very likely that, at some point in his career, the vocal artist will undergo some form of surgery. This may be surgery of the vocal folds or, more likely, an unrelated procedure, such as gallbladder surgery or a cosmetic operation. Most women will deliver children and will hopefully continue their singing careers. The increasing acceptance of cosmetic surgery, among both men and women, and the need to stay young in the performing arts arena almost mandates some form of surgical procedure in the older artist.

Given these odds, it is important that the vocal performer be aware of all his treatment options, as well as the general and specific risks of surgical procedures. In a busy career it is often difficult to block off time for surgery, and the time for recovery is also limited. Unexpected side-effects, complications or an un-planned-for extended convalescence can cost money and harm the artist's career.

Treatment options

As surgical and anaesthetic technology continues to improve, surgery is no longer a treatment of last resort. None the less, the patient with a potential surgical condition should be fully apprised of all other treatment options. A chronic sinus infection, for example, may resolve with surgery, but may also respond to long-term antibiotics, mucolytics and nasal lavage. Particularly in diseases of the upper airways, allergic tendencies should be sought and identified, since even after surgery such sensitivities will continue and must be addressed. If the condition is recurrent, such as inflammation of the gallbladder, its frequency and severity should be weighed against the possible complications of surgical removal.

If surgery is being considered, it is useful to obtain a second, and even third, opinion. Keep in mind that, while younger physicians are often more surgically inclined and older ones may be more conservative, conservatism is not invariably the better road. If there is a consensus opinion for surgery, consider all the potential benefits and complications of the procedure, and also discuss the alternative surgical techniques available for treatment. Ask specifically how experienced the surgeon is with this particular procedure, and also ask whether he has worked with singers before. While 'the latest in technology' may be available, it may not be appropriate for your condition. For example, certain lesions of the vocal folds are probably better removed with microscopic instruments than with the laser. The laser specifically has acquired a 'star wars' cachet, and somehow has come to imply atraumatic surgery, a sort of 'healing by light'. While there are specific procedures (not just in the larynx, but also elsewhere in the body), that are best treated with the laser, this technique is not a panacea. More important is the overall experience of the surgeon, which allows him to decide what instruments or technology are most appropriate.

General effects of surgery

Surgery, no matter how minor, is a form of trauma. Along with the physical aspects of the procedure, there is also the stress of anaesthesia, and the psychological stress associated with anticipation, with passive submission, and the stress of recovery which may be accompanied by pain or discomfort. The overall stress response weakens the immune system temporarily. It is not uncommon for a cold to declare itself following surgery, or for a low-grade infection to flare up. It is therefore important that the patient be as well as possible (except of course for his surgical condition) prior to undergoing a procedure. Some surgeons recommend vitamin C prior to an operation, since this seems to have a positive effect on healing. An important way to reduce stress is to have full knowledge of the procedure and its anticipated sequelae, and to have confidence in the surgeon. An informed and knowledgeable patient feels that he is part of the treatment team, rather than a passive victim of unknown and unforeseen events. A second general aspect of surgery, particularly important for the singer, is dehydration. Patients are typically asked to refrain from eating or drinking for at least 6 hours prior to surgery. They are somewhat dehydrated at the onset of the procedure, and are variably rehydrated with intravenous fluids during the procedure. Drying (anticholinergic) medications are often given at the onset of anaesthesia to reduce secretions, and further dehydrate mucous membranes. After the procedure, the patient may not be ready to drink for some time. If oxygen is given by facial or nasal mask, this further dries the upper airway.

For a singer, dryness of the vocal apparatus poses a potential problem. Although the patient will not sing for some time after convalescence, the vocal folds continue to approximate in non-vocal movements throughout the perioperative period. If an endotracheal tube is used to administer general anaesthetic, additional trauma to the vocal folds may ensue (this will be discussed further below).

While some degree of dehydration is unavoidable, singers should drink as much as comfortably possible during the day or two prior to surgery. They should also inform the anaesthetist of their concerns, and if possible ask that the use of anticholinergic medications be avoided or minimized. Following surgery small but frequent sips of water will help to moisturize the mucous membranes without distending the stomach and causing regurgitation. A third common problem after surgery is recovery of good pulmonary function. During surgery, the lungs are not fully inflated, and the cough reflex is suppressed. Following surgery, it may be uncomfortable to breathe deeply or to cough. As a result small amounts of fluid may collect in the lungs, and inflammation or even infection may follow. The options to minimize these problems are limited. With abdominal surgery, the singer should ask about endoscopic (laparoscopic) procedures. It is now possible to remove the gallbladder using a laparoscope, a steel tube that is inserted into the abdominal cavity through a small opening. This is not only less disruptive to the abdominal organs, but also minimizes cutting through the supportive muscles of the abdominal wall. The endoscope can also be used for some thoracic procedures, again minimizing trauma to the thoracic muscles.

This not only facilitates painless breathing and recovery of pulmonary function after surgery, but is also important for the singer's ability to support the voice after convalescence. The abdominal muscles (specifically the recti and the obliques) are crucial in sustaining the voice during exhalation.

Anaesthetic options

Not too long ago, a patient undergoing a surgical procedure had two options: local injection of the surgical area (similar to a dental procedure), or full general anaesthesia with laryngeal intubation. Today there are many anaesthetic options available. Specifically, for most procedures a general anaesthesia, specifically with en-dolaryngeal intubation, can be avoided. Most smaller procedures around the head and neck can be performed with a combination of local injection supplemented by intravenous sedation. The patient is rendered sleepy, and the surgical area is anaesthetized with a medication that lasts several hours. During the procedure the patient's awareness and comfort level is continuously monitored, and additional intravenous sedation is given if necessary. Most nasal and sinus procedures can be performed in this way. Operations on the middle ear, as well as cosmetic procedures on the face can also fall into this group. Tonsillectomy is an important exception: here, the anaesthetist must prevent any blood from entering the airway, and thus an endotracheal airway or laryngeal mask is used.

The combination of local or regional block with intravenous sedation is also generally used for smaller orthopaedic procedures on the extremities (such as carpal tunnel, or Dupuytren's con-tracture of the hands, or paediatric procedures), and hernia surgery. If general inhalational anaesthetic is deemed necessary, the anaesthetist may still avoid intubation by use of a laryngeal mask.

The laryngeal mask is similar in principle to a face mask ('oxygen mask'). It is smaller in size, and is placed in the back of the throat to fit over the larynx. Once in position, it is inflated and seals of the airway from the rest of the pharynx. For short procedures requiring general anaesthesia, or for patients too anxious to tolerate local anaesthesia with intravenous sedation, the laryngeal mask is a useful alternative. Specifically for the vocal artist, the laryngeal mask covers rather than invades the larynx, and minimizes trauma to the vocal folds.

Minimally traumatic intubation anaesthesia

Thus far, we have discussed surgery and anaesthesia as if we had a catalogue of options. Of course, surgery is not always optional, and there may be situations where a full general anaesthesia with endolaryngeal intubation is necessary. Like the general population, singers may be involved in accidents, develop serious or life-threatening conditions or require prolonged surgical procedures. In these instances, the need to save a life, to remove potentially fatal disease, or to correct a debilitating condition takes precedence. Once the patient understands the severity of his disease and treatment options are limited, it is generally wise to defer clinical decisions to the physician.

There are several components to a minimally traumatic intubation anaesthestic. If the patient has the opportunity he should inform the anaesthetist that he is a singer whose livelihood depends on his larynx. He should request, if possible, that should an intubation be necessary, it is performed by an experienced anaesthetist. Particularly in teaching hospitals, the intubation should be done by a qualified specialist, not a student or a trainee.

The endotracheal tube used should be the smallest one that can adequately deliver anaesthesia and protect the airway. The choice of tube size is made by the anaesthetist, and this is an area where experience is important. Although tubes of 'standard size' are generally used, for the vocalist a smaller size represents less trauma, and is therefore desirable.

Anaesthesia is usually accompanied by a paralytic agent. This allows the anaesthetist to control completely the patient's breathing, an important part of managing respiration and oxygenation. The paralysis is reversed at the end of surgery, and spontaneous breathing resumes. The tube may be removed either just before or just after spontaneous breathing movements return. Since these movements are accompanied by movements of the vocal folds, it is our suggestion that, if possible, the tube be removed before the folds begin to move. This 'deep extubation' removes the tube before the vocal folds start to come together, and minimizes trauma to their vibrating surfaces.

During extubation there may some retching, with reflux of stomach acid. Some anaesthesiologists routinely suction the stomach before awakening the patient, in order to prevent this. Along with suctioning, postoperative antinausea medications can prevent damage to the vocal folds by stomach acid. The increasing recognition of perioperative acid reflux has led some laryngologists to recommend antacid medications prior to surgery.

Once in the recovery room, the patient should be given a facial mask with humidified air or oxygen. Humidity is important, as is voice rest. Unnecessary talking, particularly in a noisy recovery room, can further traumatize the vocal folds.

Early convalescence

Even the singer cognizant of possible vocal damage will feel the need, after surgery, to cough. This cough clears the airway of secretions, and is part of the process of reinflating the lungs. If possible, coughing should be done with minimal trauma. A forceful clearing of the airway without approximating the vocal folds, or a single strong cough, is better that repeated paroxysms of coughing. If the lungs are not properly reinflating, physical therapy can help, and should be offered. Postural drainage and clapping over the chest can loosen secretions and make the cough more productive.

Pain is a frequent part of convalescence. While excessive pain should not be tolerated, the singer needs also to be aware of the side-effects of excessive analgesics. An over-sedated patient may not cough effectively, and recovery of lung function may be delayed. Some analgesics are drying, an undesirable state for the vocal performer. Medications containing codeine or codeine analogues are also constipating. Straining on the toilet involves forceful approximation of the vocal folds, and should be minimized. Indeed, if the patient is constipated for any reason following surgery, he should request a mild laxative.

When can singing be resumed? After any surgical procedure requiring endotracheal intubation, the singer should not vocalize for at least 4 to 5 days. If at that time the voice is not clear, another 5 days of rest should be considered. If after 12 days the voice is not normal, the larynx should be examined by a laryngologist to make sure there is no evidence of haemorrhage or trauma. Once the singer has a clear bill of health, full vocal activity may be resumed. Mild residual oedema may create difficulty at the top of the range, and this need not be a cause for concern. Prolonged vocal rest is to be avoided, since disuse of the larynx can create its own problems, such as atrophy. After prolonged intubation (such as may be necessary for coma after an accident), the larynx should be examined prior to any vocal exertion. Prolonged intubation can not only cause mucosal damage in the posterior part of the larynx, but can also result in malpositioning of the vocal folds. These conditions may require medical treatment and voice therapy.

Surgery of the vocal tract

The commonest operations involving the vocal tract are surgery of the nose and sinuses, removal of tonsils and surgery to the vocal folds. While these are considered minor procedures by the general population, for professional vocal artists a career may hang in the balance. Since these procedures are usually elective, the singer should consider all other options, and seek various opinions, as discussed above.

Once the decision is made to undergo surgery, the patient needs to be aware of the anticipated benefits and possible complications of the procedure. For the singer or actor, two important questions need be asked: when can he or she return to full vocal effort, and will the quality of the voice be affected by the surgery?

In cases where nasal or sinus surgery is planned, there is often persistent swelling in the nasal passage, which may last several weeks. This is normal, and usually resolves gradually. It does mean, however, that the performer may not be able to breathe freely through the nose for a while. If the obstruction was significant, even this swelling may be better than prior to surgery. After nasal septal surgery, the two upper frontal incisor teeth can lose sensation, and this may persist for several weeks. This is due to the fact that the nerves to these teeth, which run along the floor of the nostrils, have been disturbed. This condition also normally resolves over time. A common question pertains to whether the voice quality changes after surgery to the nose. The answer is no. The nose, being part of the facial skeleton, does resonate with voice production, but this is more a sensation than an acoustic phenomenon. Effective singing is done with the palate elevated, and no sound passing up through the nasopharynx. Some authors suggest that the nasal cavity may resonate due to transmitted vibrations though its floor, the hard palate. None the less, the singer feels the resonance across the face, 'the mask'. The full answer, therefore, is that, while the singer may feel a difference in resonance during singing, the actual voice produced is essentially unchanged. Further, she may enjoy an improvement in breathing efficiency due to the open nasal passages.

Removal of the tonsils in adults may help in cases of chronic recurrent infection. When the tonsils are chronically infected, any transient weakening of the immune system allows the bacteria to flourish, and the infection to flare up. Stress associated with work, personal conflicts, dieting and travel (all part of a performer's life) temporarily weakens the immune system and can lead to recurrent tonsillitis.

If for any reason chronically infected tonsils are not removed (either because the physician or the singer feels it is not wise), temporizing measures, such as topical painting of the area with antiseptic solution, or cleaning of the tonsil crypts in the outpatient department by the physician can sometimes prove helpful. Recently, ablation of the crypts with a carbon dioxide laser as an outpatient under local anaesthetic has proved helpful.

Removal of the tonsils in singers must be done carefully, to minimize scarring. The tonsils are located on either side of the soft palate, between two folds of mucous membrane-covered muscle, the 'pillars'. These pillars must be carefully preserved, and a minimal amount of mucous membrane only should be removed during surgery. Excessive excision may lead to scarring and tethering of the palate at the sides. After tonsillectomy, we encourage singers to begin exercising the palate. Even though oedema will temporarily limit the excursion of the palate, the palate should be lifted several times a day to prevent binding. This can be started even before the performer starts to vocalize.

Surgery of the vocal folds

The ultimate fear of singers, and challenge to their laryngologist, is surgery to the vocal folds themselves. For the singer, the vocal folds represent the essence of their livelihood, minute structures which bear the weight of years of training, and often physical and personal sacrifice. This understandable trepidation is fuelled by anecdotes of singers who had undergone surgery and 'were never the same after'. Some physicians, ostensibly in the name of conservatism, have gone so far as to declare that a singer should never have surgery of the vocal folds. While this fits in with the performer's natural aversion, it is wrong, and may unnecessarily condemn the performer to years of unnecessary (and unsuccessful) voice therapy, or crippling limitations to their vocal career. While vocal fold surgery should not be casually considered, it should also not be thought of as a heroic measure of last resort.

The first decision a singer must make, when vocal fold surgery has been proposed, is if it is indeed necessary. This depends, first and foremost, on the accurate diagnosis of the vocal problem. Most laryngeal conditions impairing singing have both a structural and a functional component. For example, a singer who belts or uses glottal attack excessively (problems of function) may develop nodules (structural problems). Conversely, a performer with a vocal polyp (structural) may make compensatory adjustments in technique (functional) to minimize its effects. Vocal fold cysts (structural) may cause compensatory posturing (functional) which may lead to the formation of a nodule (structural) on the opposite fold. Once the cause versus effect puzzle of structural and functional problems is unravelled, both need to be actively addressed. Voice therapy (laryngeal re-training) is an inseparable part of the treatment of any laryngeal lesion.

It is none the less clear that certain laryngeal problems must be treated surgically if they are to resolve definitively and completely. These include vascular lesions, such as varices, telangiectasia and microaneurysms resulting in recurrent haemorrhage. Laryngeal polyps, which may arise following haemorrhage or other injury, will not respond to voice therapy, and must be removed. Cysts are under the vibrating surface, and their size is not at all affected by a change in technique. By contrast, vocal fold nodules often decrease dramatically with therapy. Even if their removal is contemplated, this should not be undertaken without aggressive retraining of the phonating mechanism. Therapy in these cases serves two functions: it shrinks the nodules prior to surgery, and eliminates the faulty vocal technique which can cause recurrence following the operation.

Once the singer has come to the realization that no amount of voice rest, therapy, allergy treatment or antibiotics can bring back the voice, she should set about finding the right surgeon for this important task. We recommend obtaining several opinions. Two opinions may not agree, and the third one may cast the deciding vote. Since the problem is typically chronic, the performer should be examined on more than one occasion by the consultants. At the conclusion of these visits, a consensus of opinions usually emerges.

The techniques employed by laryngeal surgeons vary. Surgery for the singer is different from surgery for laryngeal cancer or papillomas. Be certain, therefore, to select a laryngologist who treats the performer's larynx. The treatment in most cases will involve examining the larynx with a microscope, and carefully cutting away the minute amount of excess tissue forming the polyp or nodule. Lasers may be used in some cases. They are very helpful with vascular lesions, but not essential for polyps or nodules. Do not, therefore be seduced by the 'star wars' cachet of the laser. It is just another technique for removing tissue, and it may actually be more traumatic than precise microsurgical methods.

Even if a lesion is clearly surgical, it is wise to have a voice therapist see the patient prior to surgery, to discuss postoperative management. Following surgery, the patient should be on complete voice rest for a period of up to 5 to 10 days. The duration varies with the size of the lesion removed, and the complexity of the surgery. As vocalization is resumed, the patient should start by gently stretching the cords, practising soft glissandos. Several short sessions a day (a minute or two) are recommended. Once the surface of the operated vocal fold has healed and the oedema resolved, increasingly normal vocal tasks are resumed.

Stroboscopy of the larynx both before and after surgery is helpful in monitoring the mobility of the vocal folds. A still photograph will not show stiffness or areas of decreased mobility, problems that can cause voice problems in an apparently 'normal' larynx. By monitoring the healing process, the laryngologist can better intervene to prevent possible scarring or other problems.

Suggested reading

Aronson, A. E. *Clinical Voice Disorders*, 3rd edn. Thieme Inc, New York, 1990.

Baken, R.J. *Clinical Measurement of Speech and Voice*. College Hill Publications, Little, Brown & Co., Boston, Toronto, San Diego, 1987.

Barlow, W. *The Alexander Technique*. Arrow Books, London, 1975.

Benninger, M.S., Jacobson, B.H., Johnson, A.F. *Vocal Arts Medicine*. Thieme Medical Publishing Inc, New York, 1994.

Bless, D.A., Abbs, J.H. *Vocal Fold Physiology: Contemporary Research and Clinical Issues*. College Hill Press, San Diego, 1983.

Boone, D.R., McFarlane, S.C. *The Voice and Voice Therapy*, 4th edn. Prentice Hall, Englewood Cliffs, New Jersey, 1990.

Brodnitz, F.S. *Vocal Rehabilitation*. American Academy of Ophthalmology and Otolaryngology, 1971.

Brodnitz, F. S. *Keep Your Voice Healthy*, 2nd ed. College-Hill Press, Houston, Texas, 1998.

Bunch, M. *Dynamics of the Singing Voice*, 2nd edn. Springer-Verlag, Vienna, New York, 1993.

Feldenkrais, M. *Body and Mature Behaviour*. International University, New York, 1949.

Greene, M.C.L., Mathieson, L. *The Voice and its Disorders*, 5th edn. Whurr Publishers, London, 1989.

Hammar, R.A. *Singing – An Extension of Speech*. The Scarecrow Press Inc., Metuchen, NJ, London, 1978.

Hirano, M. *Clinical Examination of the Voice*. Springer-Verlag, Vienna, New York, 1981.

Hixon, T.J. *Respiratory Function in Speech and Song*. Taylor and Francis Ltd, London, 1987.

Keidar, Anat. Personal communication, New York, 1988.

Khambata, A.S. Anatomy and physiology of voice production: the phenomenal voice. In: *Music and the Brain* (Critchley, M., Henson, R.A. eds) Heinemann Books, London, 1977.

Large, J. (ed) *Contributions of Voice Research to Singing*. College-Hill Press, Houston, Texas, 1980.

Lawrence, Van L. *Transcripts of the Thirteenth Symposium Care of the Professional Voice*. The Voice Foundation, New York, 1984.

Leyerle, W.D. *Vocal Development through Organic Imagery*, 2nd edn. College Print Shop at SUNY Genesco, 1986.

Prater, R.J., Swift, R.W. *Manual of Voice Therapy*. Little, Brown & Co., Boston, Toronto, 1984.

Proctor, D.F. *Breathing, Speech and Song*. Springer-Verlag, Vienna, New York, 1980.

Punt, N.A. *The Singer's and Actor's Throat*. Heinemann Books, London, 1979.

Reid, C.L. *A Dictionary of Vocal Terminology: an Analysis*. Joseph Patelson Music House, New York, 1983.

Rodenburg, P. *The Right to Speak*. Methuen Drama, London, 1992.

Sataloff, R.T. *Professional Voice: the Science and Art of Clinical Care*. Raven Press, New York, 1991.

Sears, T.A. Some neural and mechanical aspects of singing. In: *Music and the Brain* (Critchley, M., Henson, R.A. eds) Heinemann Books, London, 1977.

Sundberg, J. *The Science of the Singing Voice*. Northern Illinois University Press, Dekalb, Illinois, 1987.

Vennard,W. *Singing: the Mechanism and the Technic*. Carl Fischer, New York, 1967.

Winsel, R. *The Anatomy of Voice. An Illustrated Manual of Vocal Training*. Hudson House Edition, New York, 1984.

Titze, I.R., Scherer, R.C. *Vocal Fold Physiology: Biomechanics, Acoustics and Phonatory Control*. Denver Institute of Performing Arts, Denver, Colorado, 1983.

Glossary

abduct	To move away from midline.
abrupt glottal attack	(also coup de glotte, glottal stop) Build-up of air pressure beneath closed vocal folds with sudden release of air or phonation.
adduct	To move towards midline.
allergen	An agent that produces a manifestation of allergy.
amplitude	Extent of vibratory movement as in the sound wave. Measured in decibels.
androgen	A substance to stimulate or produce development of male characteristics.
anterior	Situated toward the front.
antigen	A substance which stimulates the production of antibodies or reacts to them.
aphonia	Absence of all phonation.
atrophy	Reduction in size.
bilateral	Two sided.
biopsy excision	The removal of a small piece of living tissue for microscopic examination, usually to establish a diagnosis.
bowed vocal cords	Vocal cords assume elliptical or curved form resulting in imperfect approximation during phonation.
chronic	Of extensive duration or recurring frequency.
commissure	A place where two parts join or come together.
diplophonia	Double vibration in the vocal mechanism, e.g. one vocal cord vibrates at perceivably different rate from the other cord.
distal	Far from the point of attachment.
dysphagia	Difficulty in swallowing.
dysphonia	Partial loss of phonation.
dyspnoea	Difficult or laboured breathing causing air hunger.
endoscopy	Visual examination of interior of body through natural outlets by instruments using lens systems or electric lights.
falsetto	Highest voice register.

frequency	Number of complete vibrations or cycles per second as in sound wave; measured in Hertz.
glottal chink	Small opening in the glottis.
glottis	Space between the true vocal cords.
haematoma	Focus of the blood clotting into a solid mass becoming encapsulated by connective tissue.
hyperaemic	Reddened, excessive amount of blood.
hyperfunction	Excessive use of muscular force; over tense muscle tonus.
hypernasal	Excessive nasal reconance.
hypofunction	Lack of muscular force; overly lax muscle.
hyponasality	(also closed nasality and nasality). Inadequate nasal reconance.
intubation, endotracheal	Introduction of a tube into the larynx to assume air supply, for anaesthesia.
jitter	Variations in the frequency (Hz) of a sound, usually rhythmic jitter.
laryngoscope	Instrument for direct examination of the larynx.
Lombard effect	Increasing the intensity of the voice to compensate for the masking effect of noise, music, etc.
mucosa	A mucous membrane. Membrane filled with mucus glands, lining body passages and cavities communicating outside the body.
mucus	Liquid secreted by the mucous glands.
nodules, vocal	Initially slight reddening, then localized swelling or thickening, in a mature nodule the thickening is replaced by fibrotic tissue, white or greyish in colour.
oedema	Excessive collection of fluid in tissue spaces causing swelling.
palpation	Use of hand to determine condition of body or underlying organs.
phonasthenia	Voice fatigue or weakness.
polyp	Tumour consisting of connective tissue, blood or fluid.
prognosis	The prediction of the outcome of a planned treatment procedure.
psychogenic	Originating in the mind or in emotional or mental conflict.
puberphonia	Adolescent voice.
purulent	Consisting of or forming pus.
shimmer	Variations in intensity (dB) of a sound, usually rhythmic.
stroboscope	Instrument with intermittent light source used to

give the illusion of slowing, stopping, or reverse movement.

subglottic   Below the glottis.

submucosa   The layer of areolar connective tissue under a mucous membrane.

sulcus, vocal fold   Anomaly seen as a fine longitudinal furrow on the medial edge of one or both vocal folds.

superior   Upper, towards the top.

supraclavicular   Above the level of the clavicles or collar bones.

supraglottic   Above the glottis.

tessitura   The portion of a singer's range within which production is easiest and most beautiful. Also pitch region where most notes lie for a given part.

tonsils   (also palatine or faucial tonsils). Masses of lymphoid tissue between anterior and posterior faucial pillars.

vocal fry   (also creaky). Lowest voice register; speaking in pulses at lowest possible pitch level.

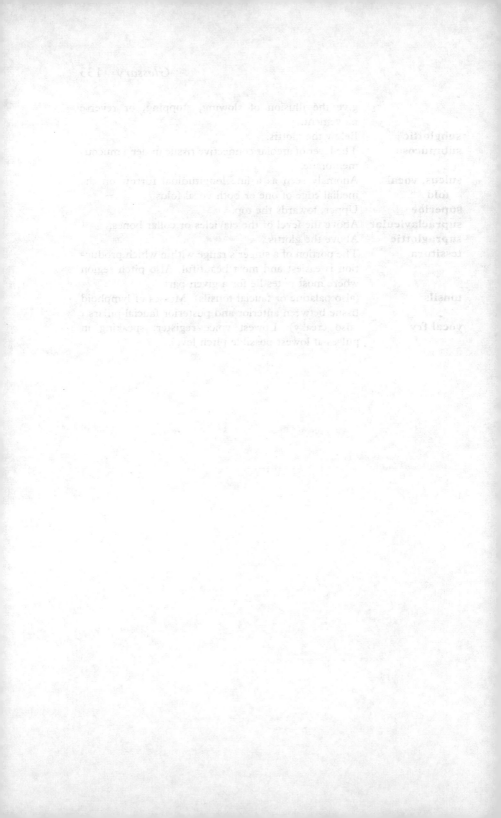

Glossary 11

simple click
subharmonics

sulcus, vocal
fold
superior
supraclavicular
suprahyoid
tessitura

tonsils

vocal fry

Index